NEVER
— TOO —
LATE

Inspiration, Motivation, and Sage
Advice from **7 Later-in-Life**
Athletes

KATE CHAMPION

Never Too Late
Inspiration, Motivation, and Sage Advice
from 7 Later-in-Life Athletes

Published by Mountain Morning Press, Ltd.
ISBN: 978-1-7344806-0-3 (paperback)
ISBN: 978-1-7344806-1-0 (ePub)
Also available for Kindle

Cover design: Vanessa Mendozzi
Layout and pre-press: Lighthouse24

Publisher's Legal Disclaimer

This book presents a wide range of opinions about a variety of topics related to physical health, mental health, diet, exercise, and general well-being including certain ideas, treatments, and procedures that may be hazardous without proper medical advice. The material presented is not intended as medical and/or healthcare advice. Please consult your healthcare provider before starting any supplements, diet, and/or exercise program. The interviewees, the author, and the publisher disclaim responsibility for any adverse effects directly or indirectly from any information contained in this book.

In loving memory of my mum. Your love of books and words continue to shine through me.

And to the Champion side of the family – the constant light through many storms.

Contents

INTRODUCTION

SO, A BIT ABOUT ME. Born in the early 1960s. I am horrible with dates and times; I think I turn 57 this year – after a while, it all runs together. I am married with two grown children. My big passion is the outdoors. If I don't get my weekly dose of the woods, I feel it: evidenced by a cranky disposition, aches and pains, and a general lack of motivation. My preferred method of movement is running, hiking, walking – anything that connects me with the earth, the pines, and that indescribable sense of stillness.

Currently, I am transitioning away from the role of motherhood toward more time on the trail and in nature. I don't buy into the socially contrived 'crisis mentality': the mid-life crisis, the quarter-life crisis, the three-quarter life crisis. I see life as a series of natural transitions. Consider womb to birth, home to school, high school to work, college to work, single to partnered, children in the home to children out of the home, periods of wellness, and periods of illness. Unfortunately, we do a great job of pathologizing the natural cycles that occur within a lifetime.

The inspiration for this project literally came to me on my way home from my first ever backpacking trip. The idea hit me like a ton of bricks so much so that I pulled the car over and scribbled down my thoughts along with a rough outline for the project. I had no clue what I was doing. But, hey – minor details.

Although I like to write, I don't consider myself a writer. Other than a couple of academic papers, I have never published anything in my life. It seems I also have a genetic predisposition for exploration and adventure. It's in my blood; probably from my mother's side of the family. As a child, I remember being mesmerized by the stories, pictures, and mementos my Great Aunt shared about her travels around the globe. In today's world my Aunt Freda would be considered quite the adventurer with her voyages across oceans and exploration of exotic lands.

I have heard my condition described as 'ants in the pants' or 'itchy feet'. I particularly resonate with the 'itchy' part of that expression. Sometimes the itch is so bad it feels like my head is going to explode. I learned recently that there is actually a term for this: wanderlust. Wanderlust, according to the *Merriam-Webster Dictionary*, is a German word comprised from *wandern* meaning 'to wander' and *lust* meaning 'desire'.

Of course, *wanderlust* is not an illness; however, I find relief knowing that it is a thing. I liken it to going to the doctor knowing there's something up but having no idea what. You talk your symptoms through, get the relevant tests, and bingo a diagnosis is slapped on you and a course of treatment is prescribed.

I also love endurance sports. There is something about people testing their limits mentally and physically that gives me a feeling I can't quite put into words. The more endurance challenges I complete the more I want to do.

So, here's where it gets sticky. I am a female in my mid-50s who loves to get outdoors. Although I have had my fair share of health challenges, I am thankful to be well and fairly fit. I eat mostly plants and whole-grains, I move regularly, and I value sleep. Over the years I have learned to say no to crap that doesn't serve me. I love epic hikes and gnarly trail runs: the heat, the mud, the distance, and the challenge. I do 'race'. I am not fast or competitive; for me, it's about getting out there, enjoying nature, and challenging myself. I'm a true back-of-the-pack athlete who is focused on showing up and completing. I can proudly say that I have never not finished a race or an endurance challenge.

Recently, my attention has expanded to include endurance backpacking: self-reliant, multi-day hikes, with everything you need on your back. In full disclosure, prior to the backpacking trip in Kentucky that birthed this book, my back had never carried more than a lightweight hydration bladder stuffed with a gel and a Chap Stick.

Additionally, my camping experience consisted of a tent pitched in the backyard with the kids, hot water, and a restroom within spitting distance. Another well-kept secret: I appear to be directionally challenged. Left or right? North or south? "Oh, the other right..." It's a running joke in our house.

As I looked around my social circles for like-minded people who also celebrate the natural world, who want to get out in the mud, go for miles, sweat their asses off, and be willing to do it all over again, there weren't many folks around. Over the past year or so, I have connected with some local hiking and running groups but didn't really find my groove there either.

When in doubt, where do you turn? The internet of course with its vast array of podcasts, YouTube channels, Facebook groups, and blogs – so many great resources. Although I am learning a lot, I found that much of the information is served from a male perspective. That said, I have found a small contingent of women in the 25 to 35 age range, who also offer perspective, inspiration, and advice for which I am grateful.

At the end of the day, I found myself wondering: where are the people like me with similar interests who are closer to my demographic? I can't be the only person struggling with this gap – right?

So, I decided to create the community I was missing. I launched a website and a Facebook page called *Back of the Pack Athlete*. Here's my purpose statement:

> *To create community and offer support. To share stories, challenges and triumphs from back-of-the-packers all over the world. To review destinations, events, and gear. To share resources, tips, and tricks. To shine the spotlight on you and your accomplishments. To celebrate and inspire. Take what you find interesting; play, notice, and report. What helps you may help others on their journey. Email me. Connect via Facebook. Check out my blog. Welcome to the community!*

My mind had been noodling on this back-of-the-pack athlete concept for some time. And, I developed a hunger to learn about backpacking. I found a beginners' backpacking trip. I bought myself a backpack for my birthday, and off I went.

The Project

As I mentioned earlier, other than a couple of academic papers, some thank-you notes, and a blog post or two – I am not a 'writer'. I have never published anything in my life. I had no expertise in this area. I had no resources, no contacts, and no clue who would even be willing to be interviewed for the book. I just knew I had to do it. I arrived home after three blissful days outdoors, before I unpacked my pack, I penned a cohesive outline for the book and fired up Google.

My first interview was with Charlene Gibson. I had listened to a podcast interview with Charlene and thought she would be perfect. At the time of writing, Charlene holds the record for the oldest British woman to summit Cho Oyu. During the show, Charlene talked about how her mountaineering journey began when she was in her late 40s. After Google-stalking Charlene, I sent her an email explaining the project and asked her for an interview. Much to my surprise, she actually responded – that was the first surprise. The second surprise were the words, "I'd love to be interviewed." I was thrilled!

Then that, "Oh, crap; now what?" moment came as the doubts started rolling around in my brain. How does this work? What questions should I ask? Do I need contracts? What about recording and copyright issues? Again, all things I knew nothing about. On a high from that great feeling of beginning creative energy, I figured out the logistics and started to look for more athletes to come alongside Charlene.

I knew I wanted to include a range of mid to later-life people from multiple sports. Within a day or so I came across Pat Gallant-Charette, the oldest woman to swim the English Channel. Although Pat had a blog, a web page, and some local news articles

I couldn't find an email address for her. However, Pat did have a Facebook presence. I took a leap and sent Pat a message via Facebook messenger. Which, as an aside, I was unfamiliar with; do I wave first? Do people even use this thing? I thought it might be fun to share some of our initial communication:

> Facebook messenger message, June 14, 2018: *Hello... my name is Kate. In researching a project I came across your name and was inspired by your story. I am creating a collection of conversations from people in their 60s+ who continue to thrive and inspire. I would love to connect, learn more about you, and highlight your story. Would you be open to talking to me...? I would be happy to share more info about the project if that would help. I look forward to hearing from you. Thank you in advance.*

To my delight Pat responded with a request for more information. After some back and forth Pat agreed. "Sure, count me in!" she said. As a side note, since our conversation, Pat has gone on to smash several other world records.

Somewhere in the back of my mind, I had been noodling on the possibility of a conversation with the woman who led the beginners' backpacking trip I attended earlier in the year. As you will learn later, Yvonne Entingh started her backpacking journey in her mid-50s. Over the last decade, Yvonne has backpacked thousands upon thousands of miles, mostly by herself. Yvonne doesn't realize this, but since that first backpacking adventure her grace, connection, and union with the natural world has been a powerful influence on my life.

Itching to go out again, I signed up for another backpacking trip with Yvonne's company. In the process I told her a bit about the project and asked if she would be interested in having a conversation. Yvonne graciously agreed. I owe a debt of gratitude to Yvonne for nurturing a belief and igniting a confidence that I can; that we can – *that we should* – get out there and live life.

Now I was on the hunt for a triathlete for the book. Preferably a female. While hiking with a friend one day, chatting about the project, she told me about a nun who competes in triathlons. Later that day, I logged back on and searched for 'triathlete nun'. I was rewarded with almost 200,000 hits. There she was in all her tanned blue-eyed glory – Sister Madonna Buder. Sister Madonna is a world champion triathlete with many accolades under her belt. At 87 years old, she holds the record for the oldest Ironman competitor ever! I know I set the bar high with my hopes of connecting with this remarkable woman; regardless, I had to try.

How do you connect with nuns? Do nuns have email? Laptops? Access to the internet? After some digging, I was able to find an email address that I hoped was somehow connected to Sister Madonna. I sent her a carefully crafted email about the project... silence.

Then, out of the blue, about six weeks later an email from Sister Madonna popped up in my inbox. I nearly peed my pants. Sister Madonna agreed to an interview! I seriously could not believe it – we arranged a conversation for July.

Since the inception of this project I have learned much about writing, the writing process, and the ebbs and flow of creative energy. I now know there is a beginning energy. That is the good stuff: excitement, motivation, drive, joy. Then comes, what some call, the 'saggy middle'. For me, that's when those juicy feelings of excitement and motivation morph, seemingly overnight, into doubt, negativity, and what I can best describe as drudgery. What's more, this lovely array of feelings seems to be in cahoots with a cascade of annoying thoughts such as, "What am I doing?" "Really, who gives a crap?", with a grand finale, of, "No one's going to read this s**t."

If you are thinking, "Geez, this gal knows a lot about thoughts and feelings" you would be right. I am a mental health professional. That's how I earn a living. I work with people from all walks of life with an array of stuff from addictions, to trauma, to anxiety, to grief and loss. Consequently, I know a lot about 'stinking thinking'; my own, and others.

During this saggy phase, I was able to cut through the unhelpful mental chatter and remind myself that thoughts are not facts. I allowed myself a moment to wallow, then swiftly kicked myself in the rear end and told myself to 'get on with it'. Honestly, on reflection, and post whining, all these amazing conversations just fell into place, frankly pretty effortlessly.

By mid-summer, opportunities for conversations were dwindling. I wanted a male endurance runner to join the line-up. I had no leads. Sadly, the few people I found on the web, on further investigation, had passed away. That's when I went to Facebook again.

By then I had built a bit of a Facebook community. I did a 'wanted' post in a couple of the running groups I belong to. That's how I met Butch, Annie, and Dan. The universe outshone herself. There could not have three more perfect people for the project.

'Butch' (Richard Britton) started running later in life and competes in ultras at the 50K, 100K, and 100-mile distance. Annie (Annie Crispino-Taylor), also an endurance athlete, started running 5Ks in her 40s. Since then Annie has completed one 100-mile race every year from the age of 50 to 60 years old. Furthermore, during this period Annie was diagnosed with, and overcame, cancer. And Dan (Dan Taylor) is a true road warrior, who, at 85, still runs every day. In my eyes, Dan is a legend. Speaking with Dan felt like speaking with an esteemed grandfather of running, his knowledge and experience spans almost 50 years. Dan's 'fitness plan' includes running two marathons a year.

In a matter of months, I had connected with seven inspirational athletes; all so generous in their willingness to share their time and their incredible stories. Many things amazed me during this process. One thing that really stands out is that these extraordinary athletes didn't have boring, run of the mill, grayscale stories, they had amazing vibrant stories full of grit, determination, and passion. Collectively, they shared openly about cancer, PTSD, fear, loss, grief, depression, aging, spirituality, along with the joys and richness their sport has brought to their lives.

Ultimately, my hope is that this book inspires, educates, motivates, and connects people. Yet, to be completely transparent, this project also filled a selfish need. I wanted to know what's in the secret sauce. How do I stay fit, active, healthy and still rockin' into my 60s, 70s, and beyond?

A Bit about the Process

As I started to think about what I wanted to learn, I also wondered what would be helpful for other people in the same boat – they had to be out there, right? I did a bit of research and decided to go back to my trusted Facebook groups. Here's my post:

Question: If you could ask a masters plus athlete – someone in their 60s, 70s, and 80s who's still rockin' their sport anything – what would you want to know?

The majority of Facebook responders were interested in diet, training, prevention, and recovery from injuries. I wondered about their backstories, how do they deal with 'stinking thinking', and what had inspired them along the way. After some tweaking, consulting my qualitative research books – I knew they would come in handy someday – and reading other authors who have used a similar format (like Tim Ferris), I landed on 10 questions.

Not everything in the following pages will resonate with everyone. The neat thing is that you can pick and choose how, when, and where you consume these words. Take what you need and leave the rest.

Another cool thing about words is that once they are laid down, there they sit, suspended in time, patiently waiting, ready to serve whenever the mood strikes. I believe books are a gift. There is magic in handing a book to another human being, looking them in the eyes, and saying, "Here, read this, it might help…"

Final Business

- The order of questions were the same for each athlete.

- I love quotes. There are quotes scattered throughout this book. You will find quotes from the world at large, personal favorites from the athletes, along with quotes that resonated with me from our conversations.

- Each conversation has gone through an editing process simply to help with flow and readability.

- You are getting 95% of what I got from the interviewees. If I didn't get an answer, you'll know that too.

- The chapter on motivations and beliefs is framed from my education, practice, and training as a mental health professional.

- In the back of the book you will find resources and an index. These sections include the books, races, trails, etc. – with links where possible – that the athletes mention. Plus, other stuff I have found helpful along the way.

- There's also a note of thanks. Gratitude is a value of mine.

- Lastly, stop by the *final words* page and re-member to follow katechampionauthor.com so you can keep your eye out for other books in the series.

CHARLENE GIBSON

The oldest British woman to summit Cho Oyu

*"I know people can't always do things at the
drop of a hat, but if you set yourself a time
limit, make a plan, and tell yourself, 'Right, I'm
going to do this,' then you'll get there."*
– Charlene Gibson

CHARLENE IS A 55-YEAR-YOUNG Scottish woman who
found her passion for exploration in her mid-30s.
Charlene's quest for adventure started with trips to
Turkey and Morocco, which led to more challenging
trips to places like India and Peru. Charlene's
athletic résumé includes driving from Plymouth in
the United Kingdom to Dakar, Senegal, in a car
worth 100 British pounds (approximately $130) and
a cycling trip covering the approximately 1,000
kilometers (620 miles) between Lhasa in Tibet to
Nepal's Kathmandu.

With each trip, Charlene gained more strength
and confidence. As her confidence grew, her
appetite for mountaineering blossomed. In 2013,
Charlene decided to put her confidence to the test.
She booked a trip to climb Nepal's Mera Peak
mountain. Mera Peak is classified as a trekking

peak, which basically means a person can walk it. After successfully summiting, Charlene realized that if she wanted to get serious (and safer) about mountaineering, she had better advance her skills and knowledge.

With the big 5-0 looming closer, Charlene knew she wanted more out of life – be careful what you wish for. In celebration of her fifth decade, Charlene set her sights on summiting Cho Oyu, the sixth highest mountain in the world measuring 8,188 meters (26,863 feet) above sea level. The mountain stands majestically on the China-Nepal border. At the time of writing Charlene is the oldest British woman to summit Cho Oyu.

I am excited to share more about this incredible woman. This conversation takes a dive into what makes Charlene tick, how she works through challenges and celebrates joys. She discusses discrimination, motivation, and inspiration. Charlene also has sage advice for others wanting to strike out and make their mark on the world. Charlene, I am forever grateful. Thank-you!

Charlene G

What is your favorite quote or saying?

I actually don't have one…I have never gone down that road. I see quotes that appeal to me here and there, but there's nothing that really sticks with me.

Can you think of a book that stands out in your mind as an influential 'must read'?

I'm an avid reader. So, there are quite a few. When I was growing up, the books that influenced me the most were Enid Blyton's *The Famous Five* series. I loved all the adventures they had. I'm an only child. I grew up in a very rough area, so I didn't get outside and play with other kids much. My mum worked hard to protect me. She encouraged me to focus on doing well in school. Because I wasn't out in the neighborhood playing with other kids, reading became my entertainment. I'd read *The Famous Five*. I read *The Hardy Boys* books. I loved books with a bit of excitement, a bit of drama, and a sense of adventure. In more recent years, I've started reading again. I love biographies and I love stories about mountaineering. The books I find inspirational tell stories that leave me thinking, "I could never do that."

My mum, bless her, is at that age where she likes to go and ferret around in charity shops. She and her friends pick up mountaineering books for me. I don't think she's ever given me a book with a happy ending; there's always death in there somewhere. Over the years, my mum has given me numerous mountaineering books.

The books I have read recently include *Annapurna*, which is the story of the first conquest of an 8,000-meter peak in the Himalayas written by

French climber Maurice Herzog. Herzog was the leader of the 1950 French Annapurna expedition, the first group of mountaineers in history to summit and return from an 8,000-meter mountain. The book shares the gripping tale of their epic adventure. Be warned, it's is a difficult book to put down.

The White Spider by Heinrich Harrer is another book I would recommend. Although very exciting, the book is also factual, with vivid detail about the first ascent of the north face of the Eiger. Tom Patey's *One Man's Mountains* is another great read. He presents a collection of stories and prose about climbing. Patey was a doctor, a writer, and a prolific climber. A man with no airs and graces who had a true love for climbing. I find accounts about people who actually go out and do these incredible things hugely inspirational.

Please share a bit about your background. How did you get interested in this sport, and what were some of your first steps?

Basically, I was raised by my mum and my nana, my mum's mum. My father left us when I was three. Just got up and walked out. My mum who was 27 at the time was left to care for a toddler. Alone, with no support, she went back home to live with her mother. That was it. She's lived there ever since. She's still in that same house today. The neighborhood hasn't changed much either – it's still a very rough area. It's sad. Even now, I hear about all the crime and see kids going in and out of prison.

Although my mum went to high school, like many kids, she didn't apply herself. She had dreams of qualifying as a nurse but left nursing school two months before her final exams with her dreams unfulfilled. Instead, she married my dad and had me; that's just what you did back then. My mum was determined; she didn't want me to follow in her footsteps. She wanted me to make something out of my life.

Understandably, growing up, there was a strong focus on doing well in school. Being an only child, I didn't mix much with other kids. Understanding the importance of socialization, my mum packed me off to dancing lessons. As a kid, I danced for seven or eight years. I did tap and modern stage dancing – this is a brilliant way to get a child to come out of their shell! When I was seven years old, I started playing the bagpipes. I played the bagpipes until I was 21. Growing up, my mum was always there, behind the scenes, encouraging me and making sure I did good. I went to the Dundee College of Technology, got a degree in maths and physics. After college, I joined the Civil Service as a government employee.

Growing up, I wasn't interested in the outdoors. It just wasn't for me. Our holidays were pretty tame; nothing too adventurous. We never went abroad or anything like that. I really didn't get outdoors much until I was in my early 20s. At that time, I had a boyfriend, David. David was a keen cyclist and an outdoors guy. He introduced me to cycling. We did quite a bit of mountain biking together. We'd go off and do some camping and cycle touring, things like that.

After 12 years together, David and I parted ways. The break-up was just before Christmas. I was dreading the thought of spending Christmas and the new year on my own. I was in a rut. I knew, deep down, I wanted to do something different, something big.

I'd heard about a couple of adventure companies. So, I did a bit of research and booked an Explore holiday – two weeks trekking in Morocco. It was absolutely nerve-wracking. I'd never done anything like that before, going to as exotic a place as North Africa. I was heading out on my first big adventure completely on my own with a bunch of people I had never met. I felt like I was literally going headfirst into the unknown.

When I arrived in Morocco, it was a real shock to the system. Of course, I had camped before. However, the camping I had done always had some form of bathroom facilities. They might be pretty basic, but at the minimum you could count on a toilet block or some kind of latrine. To my horror there was nothing. The bathroom instructions were 'go and find yourself a nice rock, squat down, and hope nobody comes around the corner while you are doing your business'.

I clearly remember thinking, "I'm not sure I can do this." I quickly got used to the lack of privacy. By the end of the trip, I was totally fine with it. Now, looking back, I really enjoyed the challenge. I remember wishing I had done something like this a lot earlier in my life.

As soon as I got back home, I was hungry for another adventure. I wanted to test my limits, push myself harder. I quickly booked another trekking holiday in the Taurus Mountains in Turkey.

My goal was to keep building my strength and confidence by finding harder and harder adventures. In fact, I became a bit of a trekking snob; each time the next trek had to be harder and more challenging. I went back to Morocco. I trekked in Kazakhstan – that was amazing. I went to India, Peru, and back to Turkey to climb Mount Ararat. Each trek was getting harder and harder. The next logical step was to try a bit of mountaineering.

In 2013, I decided I would try to summit Mera Peak in Nepal. This was my first foray into mountaineering. Honestly, it was more by luck than judgement that I managed to get up to the summit of Mera Peak and back without any mishaps. This experience made me realize two things: one, that I knew nothing about mountaineering, and two, how important it is to know what I am doing.

So, that's it. I have just gone on from there. Taking small steps. Building skills and stamina. I have done bits of climbing in Scotland. I'm not somebody who tends to pack their bag and goes off by themselves. I choose commercial expeditions. I like having the security of knowing if the proverbial does hit the fan, I am not by myself.

On my trips, I was fortunate to have tour leaders who were excellent alpinists. The Mera Peak trip, for example, is sold by travel companies as a trekking peak. The peak is almost 6,500 meters high. Mera Peak can be a very cold mountain and frostbite is not uncommon. People can get lulled into a false sense of security. It's easy to think, "A trekking peak? How difficult can that be?" On our trip, we all did well. Out of six people, five of us actually summited the peak.

In retrospect, the thing I found most challenging was not knowing what I was doing. Because I didn't have the experience, I didn't feel confident or particularly safe. Honestly, if anything had happened, I wouldn't have known what to do. I didn't want to put myself in that position again. After that trip, I decided to take more advanced courses. When I got home, I signed up for a mountaineering course with the International School of Mountaineering (ISM). These courses helped immensely to hone my skills and build confidence.

As my birthday approached, I wanted to do something epic to celebrate my fiftieth year. My thoughts were pulling me toward climbing Cho Oyu. Another thing that spurred my decision was the news that a close friend was diagnosed with terminal brain cancer. He was 42. The news was a real shock. He was a big strapping bloke, 6-foot-5. He looked perfectly healthy. I know you can't tell who's going to succumb to illness and who isn't. With him, you would never have known. The doctors said he had somewhere between six months and five years to live. Until he got that diagnosis, his life had just been trundling along quite happily. He was a good man doing his best to take care of himself and his family. You don't imagine that suddenly your whole world can come crashing down around you.

The news of his diagnosis struck me deeply. I knew that if I'm going to do something, then I had better do it now. I'm like a lot of people. You think, "Oh, I'll do that at someday," or "I can't be bothered to do that just now." The thought of my young healthy friend facing the end of his life really pushed me. I felt a sense of urgency. I needed to do something soon. There's absolutely no guarantee that you'll get that 'one day'. So, I booked the trip.

I knew Cho Oyu was way beyond my comfort zone. It didn't matter. I wanted to do something really memorable. I booked the trip with a chap I had met on the Mera Peak trip, Rolfe Oostra. Rolfe owns the adventure company called 360 Expeditions. I liked the way he guided, and I liked his attitude.

I did more alpine courses with ISM. I wanted to make sure I was completely happy with stretching myself and learning top-notch mountaineering skills. After three intense weeks of training in Switzerland, I came home absolutely shattered. On the plus side, my crevasse rescuing was second to none. These intensive courses made a huge difference in my skill and confidence level.

Coincidently, around the same time a couple of people at work who were in my age range, or younger, received cancer diagnoses. Sadly, within the year, both people had died. Again, another massive hit over the head: do not put things off because there's no guarantee that you will be afforded the opportunity to actually do those things. This spurred me on even more. It's a shame that it takes something like this to really bring home the fact that life is short; better late than never, I suppose.

I think it's the fact that we assume that everything's going to be fine because stuff happens to other people. Or maybe we think that this happens to old people. We forget, or don't realize, that we are getting older, too.

In reality, I am now older than my nana was when I was born. To me, as a kid, my nana always looked old. Yet, I look at myself and I think, well, I'm not old. I'm only 52, I'm not old. Of course, I am getting older. Again, there's no guarantee that everything will continue to go well.

Tell me about some of the joys, challenges, and milestones along the way.

One of the most stunning trips I recall was the trip to Kazakhstan. This trip was full of life lessons. My main bag went missing; so much of my kit didn't make it to our destination. Fortunately, for the first time ever, I split-packed a little bit. Thankfully, I had worn my boots. I always wear my boots on the plane; that's the one thing that you really don't want to be without. I also had a few bits and pieces [of equipment with me] and managed to buy some odds and ends to tide me over. I begged and borrowed stuff from other people. Pretty soon, I had enough gear to make do. This experience taught me two lessons: one, I realized the importance of making sure I keep the important items on my person (nowadays, it's not unusual for me to wear all my mountaineering gear on the plane); and two, it's amazing what you can do without – my bag finally turned up.

We spent 10 days trekking in the Tian Shan mountains. Another learning from that trip was realizing that I'm not a natural horse rider. We rode pack mules for about 15 kilometers (approximate nine miles). Riding those pack mules is probably one of the most uncomfortable experiences of my life, ever!

The Tian Shan mountains were absolutely beautiful. First off, you had the classic alpine experience. After that, we flew up to the South Inylchek Glacier and trekked. Here you have mountains. You've got

Khan Tengri on one side and Pobeda up there, too. This was the most stunning place that I have ever seen. We flew up in this big Russian helicopter specially equipped to fly at high altitudes. Once we were dropped off in the camp, we were surrounded by nothing except big, white, pointy mountains. From our camp, we trekked toward Pobeda one day. This was a memorable moment because this was such a different experience for me compared to my previous trips. To this day, I have never, ever seen scenery like it. It was absolutely beautiful.

In 2009, I cycled from Lhasa to Kathmandu. This was another memorable experience. I'd never been to Tibet before. I'd read a book called *My Journey to Lhasa* by Alexandra David-Néel. The book, set in the early 20th century, is a memoir about a European explorer who disguised herself as a Tibetan woman. Alexandra spoke fluent Tibetan. She entered and then lived in Tibet during a time where foreigners were forbidden. The story narrates the author's lived experience in Lhasa before being discovered. It was this story about her incredible adventure that sparked my desire to visit to Lhasa.

We cycled along the Friendship Highway, detouring along the way to visit Everest northern base camp and headed up toward the tourist part. Everest looks absolutely stunning from this direction. Because of the angle, the mountain looks as if it's actually on its own. When you're accessing the mountain from the Nepal side, Everest gets almost dwarfed with Ltohse, the fourth highest mountain on one side, and Luptse on the other. Everest doesn't stand out like you think it would. But, when viewed from the Tibetan side, Everest looks absolutely incredible.

Of course, the real highlight for me so far, the thing I have bored everyone to death with, is climbing Cho Oyu in 2016 – that was so amazing. Cho Oyu is a nice-looking mountain. Cho Oyu, located in Tibet, is the sixth highest mountain in the world at 8,201 meters. To get there, we flew up to Lhasa from Kathmandu then traveled in a minibus. Lhasa has grown hugely since I was last there in 2009. We then stayed at Shigatze for a couple of nights. Shigatze is another city that has grown a lot. Along the way, we stopped at a village called Tingri, which has changed, for the better, over the last decade. You can see how the investments in new schools and other infrastructure have benefitted these small villages.

When you arrive to climb Cho Oyu, the first step is to check in at the Chinese base camp. From there, we moved up to an interim camp, then on to advanced base camp. As you can imagine, there is an acclimatization process which takes a while. We spent close to six weeks at advanced base camp surrounded by the most superb scenery. The mountains are sitting there right in front of you. The whole time, you're surrounded by this incredible snowy, majestic beauty. It's absolutely lovely.

I like base camp life. Obviously, at that elevation, there is no mobile phone signal. Everest base camp is a bit different; they do have all the mod cons [modern conveniences]. On Cho Oyu, there's nothing. No mobile phone signal, no internet, no nothing. You're completely cut off from the world, which I really enjoyed. There's nothing to do apart from eat, sleep, and sleep some more. You do a bit of washing. You sit around. On this trip, there were three small teams sharing the same facilities. On our team, team 360, we had five people: myself, my friend Kam, Alex, Arthur, and Rolfe who was our guide. There were also five people in the other group.

We had five climbing Sherpas supporting us. They were fantastic. Between them, they had something like 56 Everest summits. Everyone was so helpful and friendly. Just amazing people. Everyone got along really well. Camp life is nice. You sit there. You have a chat. You play cards. You go to your tent. You read a book. You don't have to worry about anything at all.

Thinking about food as fuel, what have you tried diet-wise? What has been helpful? Are there any supplements you swear by? Do you have any must-have foods when training or competing? What is a treat in your world?

When it comes to food, I don't have any preferences at all. During the summer, I like salads. My salads consist of spinach leaves and a variety of other stuff. I'm not vegetarian or anything like that. I don't eat anything special. I am not much of a cook; it's not something I enjoy. I like to make things that are easy. I like couscous because it's quick and simple. I prefer simple, real food ingredients, things that I can just throw into a pan. An example of a quick, simple meal would be some couscous with cherry tomatoes, sweet peppers, mushrooms, and a chicken breast. That's fine for me.

I don't worry too much about my diet. Honestly, at times, my diet can be absolutely dreadful. Particularly when I am short on time. I remember trying to complete my final writing assignment for my degree. Because I'm inherently lazy, I leave things to the last minute; I like to think I work best under pressure. During that time, my diet literally consisted of crisps [potato chips] and chocolate. I'd rip right through them. I try not to do that too much. I don't take any supplements either. I am not particularly great when it comes to food.

Like I said, I'm not much of a foodie. I do like nuts and things like that. Again, it's food that's easy. I must have chocolate. When I'm out training, doing hills or climbs, I tend not to eat enough, so I do have to be careful about getting enough calories.

On the mountain, once we were out at advanced

base camp, we had to cook for ourselves, with boil-in-the-bag stuff. The food was all pre-cooked. All I had to do was warm it up. It's all about trying to get enough calories in. Ideally, if I can get enough calories in as easily as possible without having to eat a huge amount of food then that suits me a lot better.

Needless to say, a treat for me is chocolate. I eat quite a bit of chocolate. Chocolate always goes down so well. I remember sorting out all the rations before we headed out to do our rotations at base camp and making double sure there was enough chocolate to tide us over.

How did you begin to build your fitness? What were some of your early steps? And how did you know you were starting to form a habit?

The best thing I did was to hire a personal trainer. A woman and fellow mountaineer recommended a local guy she had been training with for a couple of years. I trained with him for about 10 weeks before I was scheduled to climb Cho Oyu. He made such a difference. I was going twice a week. It's not cheap by any stretch. Training with him, I felt a huge difference in my strength and stamina.

I also run and walk a lot. I tried to get as much time on my feet as possible. I'd load up my pack and off I'd go. I started small and built up to carrying about 15 kilograms (about 33 pounds). The walking, the running, and the personal training – it all helped.

It wasn't until I arrived and faced that 8,000-meter peak that I began to realize exactly what climbing an 8,000-meter peak entailed. Honestly, despite all that training, I began to wonder if I was fit or strong enough for the challenge. It's very difficult to know how it's going to feel when you are facing something for the first time. I had climbed to 6,500 meters before. I handled that well, but this was a big step up.

I was using supplemental oxygen. Although the extra oxygen helped, it's not enough to make it seem like you're walking at sea level. Getting a personal trainer and making sure I had enough time on my feet was the best thing I could have done to prepare for the climb.

I like to vary my training. On Tuesdays and Thursdays, I had my personal training sessions. He would have me doing split squats, front elevated foot squats, rear foot elevated split squats, normal squats, goblet squats, hamstring curls, and lunges. The focus was on building strength in my legs. With all the muscle growth, my legs quickly began to change shape. That was cool. We also worked hard on my upper body strength: lots of pull downs, dumbbell work, and shoulder presses.

My trainer was very good at making sure I did everything with proper form. On and off, over the years, I have gone to the gym. I've done a bit of this and a bit of that. Sometimes, I would spend an hour or an hour and a half at the gym and not accomplish very much. With the trainer, the training was so focused I was in and out in half an hour. In those 30 minutes, I worked harder, targeted more areas of my body, and saw better results than I ever did with an hour in the gym by myself. I still train with him. To keep the cost down, I started training with a small group. I have to switch my days up a bit but still train twice a week. Still doing lots of squats!

On the weekends, I pack up my bag and go for a walk. I've got woods not far from here and like-minded people to connect with. Sometimes, I meet up with other members of the Wessex Mountain-eering Club. My training plan for my expeditions include a combination of personal training, running, and steep hill work with a full pack.

Do you have any morning or evening routines?

I am a go-with-the flow person. I'm not good in the mornings. Mornings have been worse for me over the last six months or so because I've started to go through menopause. Honestly, this menopause thing has been absolutely killing me. I've been to the doctor and started hormone replacement therapy. I'm waiting to see if that will help.

As for training, I do my training in the afternoon and the evening. There's a climbing wall close to my house. I'll head over there after work. Generally, there are a couple of mates I can climb with; it all helps with the training.

My favorite time of year for running is the winter. I love heading out to the woods in the dark with a headlamp on. At night, you get to see so much more wildlife. Plus, heading out at night you have the trail all to yourself. When you're running in the light of a headlamp, as you glance to the left or the right, you see all these little eyes looking at you. I've seen deer and badgers; and, at times, heard the swoosh of owls sweeping over my head. I've also been scared to death by pheasants startling me when they suddenly fly out of the bushes. It's absolutely lovely.

Discrimination and/or negativity as an older athlete – do you think this is a thing? Have you personally experienced it? How did you deal with it? What would you tell others?

Honestly, I personally haven't experienced any discrimination. However, I do think it's a thing. It's possible I haven't experienced any discrimination because of my level in the sport. Let's face it, I'm never going to be winning any awards or anything. I am not in it for the competition. I know it sounds like I've done a lot. It's important to remember that my experiences have been spread out over a number of years. When I talk to people about the things I've done, it can sound like I'm out here every weekend scaling mountains and fighting crocodiles. This isn't the case at all.

People I've encountered on expeditions have been very supportive. On Cho Oyu, there were a lot of experienced mountaineers; people that have climbed the north face of the Eiger and been up to K2. People I have seen on TV or read about in books. In fact, we arrived in Kathmandu a bit earlier than anticipated, and we ended up partying with these guys for a couple of days. These experienced mountaineers who have done so much were absolutely chuffed to bits for our summits and so very supportive.

There's been none of this "You've not really done anything. What big mountains have you climbed?" attitude. I was actually very surprised. I assumed that the world-class mountaineers alongside us might sneer, "Half-baked amateurs, who do they think they are?" but it wasn't like that at all. Everybody was great. On reflection, I think it was the people that made that expedition such a special experience. I still keep in contact with many of them. We follow each other on Twitter, exchange text messages and the like. Not only did I summit, I feel like I made some pretty good friends along the way.

That said, I know discrimination does exist. My friend, not so much as an older athlete, but a woman also on the Cho Oyu expedition, experienced some discrimination. Like the rest of us, this woman hadn't washed her hair for six weeks. In our summit picture, my hair looked like a mess of matted felt, and her hair looked like she just stepped out of a salon. I can assure you my hair did not self-cleanse in that six-week period. But her summit picture looked amazing. My friend experienced some negative comments because she looked 'too glamorous for the mountains'. I am not perceived as 'glamorous' so I don't get these sorts of comments. So, yes, negativity and discrimination can be a thing; I've been fortunate that it's bypassed me.

We all have thoughts that can be negative: fears, doubts, that critical voice that might say, "Who do you think you are?" or "What are you thinking? You can't do that." What are some tips and tricks you use to combat your own 'stinking thinking'?

Yes, I know those negative voices. I got them on Cho Oyu. When I found it difficult to acclimatize, those negative voices really kicked in. It took me two attempts to get to camp one, and it took me two attempts to get to camp two. After I aborted my attempt to reach camp two, I remember thinking to myself, "This really is not boding well for me." I began to doubt that I would, or could, summit. I felt pretty down about the whole experience.

The following morning, Rolfe and I headed off again to see if I could get up there. In the space of an hour and a half, we covered the same distance that it had taken us four hours to do the day before. I think

I needed that extra day. We didn't have a particularly aggressive acclimatization schedule. Maybe I didn't acclimatize as quickly as everyone else.

I'll never forget arriving at camp after a failed summit attempt watching everyone else going for their summit push. That feeling of hanging back and having to wait for another chance the following evening. I vividly recall waking up the night of my summit push thinking that I could quite happily stay in my tent and not go anywhere. I didn't have my sleeping bag as I would be sleeping in my down clothing (to save weight). Regardless, my negative thoughts continued to try and convince me that I would be much happier staying in my tent. Outside, it was dark. It was cold. It was half past 10 at night, and our plan was to climb through the night and summit in the morning.

What drove away those negative thoughts was thinking about Rolfe and one of our climbing Sherpas, Padawa. These guys had summited the day before. They got back out of their beds that night to give me a chance to summit – that's what kept me going. I told myself that while I'm able to stand on my own two feet and move one foot in front of the other, there was absolutely no excuse for me to give up. That's the way I got up that mountain.

Thinking back on it, I realized I was having some really weird thoughts. My thoughts seemed to make sense at the time, but on reflection, honestly, I'm not so sure. I can't say they were exactly hallucinations but certainly bizarre thoughts that kept looping around and around as I kept trudging up higher and higher. I just kept telling myself that these people had faith in me; they were confident that I could make it up to the summit and handle the descent. I wasn't going to let them down.

I get negative around other stuff as well. Running is a good example. I know I should go for a run, but my thoughts tell me that I really can't be bothered. Then the back-and-forth starts in my head between the part that says you really should get out there and the part that says you just can't be bothered.

One thing that really spurs me on is walking to the supermarket on a Saturday morning. As I walk through the store, I see people riding mobility scooters or in wheelchairs. Or simply elderly folk doing their best to move through the town, maybe using a cane or a walker. And I'm sitting there thinking to myself, "I can't be bothered to go for a run!"

There are probably quite a few of these people who would give their eyeteeth to be able to have the opportunity to get out there for a run. And there I am, capable of running but just can't be bothered. That's the sort of thing that gives me a sharp slap on the back of the head. It's a reminder to get on with it rather than just sitting around being lazy. I'll give myself a good talking to, and say, "Right, just go and do it now. Stop putting it off."

Sometimes, I have to bargain with myself. "OK, just get your shoes on and go out there for five minutes. You'll feel better once you get out." Before you know it, I am two or three miles into the run and thinking, "Huh, I'm actually quite enjoying this now." Then I'll get back and find myself thinking that was really good. I really enjoyed it. If I'm lucky I'll get to see an owl or a falcon – something that makes it all worth it.

Then there are other days when you go out there and the whole run just feels like a slog, but even so, I'll get back and think, "Right, that was awful. I hated every single step of that," but I still feel good because I did it. Even though I didn't enjoy it, or it wasn't great I still pushed through. I have learned that it doesn't matter if the run was enjoyable or not, there's always something positive to take away from it.

Injuries & illness – have you had any major setbacks health-wise? How do you cope with injuries? Do you do anything to avoid injuries? What tips do you have for healing and recovery?

Oh, dear God, injuries, yes. I've had quite a few. Many years ago, I was at a fitness class. I won't bore you with the details of whatever exercises we were doing, but I basically tripped over my own feet and fell over. I ended up damaging the ligaments in my ankle. I managed to make it home that night. In the morning, it was so bad I had to call a friend to take me to the hospital. I thought I had broken my ankle. I couldn't put any weight on it, let alone walk on it.

The hospital put me straight into a wheelchair and started a battery of X-rays. The doctors quickly determined that my ankle wasn't broken. They promptly heaved me out of the wheelchair and handed me a Truegrip bandage, with the discharge instructions: "Right, here you go. Walk on it as much as you can." Five weeks later I still couldn't walk on it properly, so I went to another doctor who was worse than useless. He looked at it. Gave it a bit of a poke and a prod and said, "Oh, that may be as good as it gets."

Thankfully, there was a chap at work who had a similar injury a couple of months before mine. Even though it was ligament damage, he ended up in a cast. Taking my friend's advice, I made an appointment with the same physio [physical therapist]. This guy was great! He was an ex-dockyard worker with the strongest fingers I had ever seen. I saw him regularly for close to three months. He ended up smoothing out all the fibers in the tendons. He did an excellent job. During the healing process, I added some swimming and did some other strength training. After about six months, I was able to go out and do a little bit of running, as long as I was careful not to wrench or twist it. It took about two years for my ankle to feel completely normal.

My relationship with running did not develop until I was in my early 40s. When I got back from India, I realized how much running helped with building trekking endurance. As a child, I never enjoyed running, mostly because I was useless at it. I'm a bit of loner, so I joined a local running club. I found that I really enjoyed running and the social aspect of it. Pretty soon, Wednesday nights became running night. A group of us would head out and run the streets of Salisbury. I made some good friends along the way.

Anyway, I started running more and more. I even did a couple of races. I started to notice some little niggles in my Achilles tendon. Nothing seemed too serious, so I just ignored it. During training for a 20-mile run, one day as I was helping to move something at work (my job can be pretty physical), I felt a funny feeling under my knee. Anyway, I didn't think any more of it. I felt that same sensation a couple more times during that week. Pretty soon, the sensation crept to the outside of my ankle and up through my leg. Again, I just ignored it.

Well, I did the 20-mile run, but the upshot was that I had a stress fracture in my leg. So off to the hospital I go again. They said, "Well, there's nothing we can really do. You just need to rest it." That knocked me back a bit. I was overtraining and ignoring what my body was trying to tell me. Through overtraining, I also ended up having lesions in one of my Achilles tendons and was off running for a year.

More recently, I began climbing with a chap. Although we started out at a similar skill level, I noticed he was quickly getting better than me. In reaction to the competition I decided to push myself a bit more. I ended up overdoing it and developed tennis elbow. Another injury that has taken about six months to heal.

A lot of the time my injuries come from over-training. I also think part of my problem is that I am not realizing that I am getting older. I need to slow down a bit and be more careful about what I am doing. Maybe not go hell for leather so much, but actually do things like stretching, warming up, and cooling down – all things I *should* be doing.

This is where my personal trainer helps. His goal is to make me injury proof by building up everything in my body. He's all about maximizing the mobility in all your joints. It's helped me a lot with my shoulders and hips. With the stretching, warming up, cooling down, and listening to my body, I am hopeful that I'll be able to keep injuries at bay.

I'd love to hear about what inspires you... Who are your role models? How do you stay motivated?

When I look back, there's so much stuff I wish I'd done when I was younger. For instance, I wish I had taken a year off and gone traveling. At times, I wish I'd started doing outdoor stuff sooner, but in reality, at that time, I just wasn't interested. So, part of my motivation comes from the fact that I am getting older.

My mum is hugely inspiring to me. She sacrificed so much to give me the best possible start in life. She supported me. She made sure that I stuck with school. She always encouraged me to do my best. Although I didn't appreciate it at the time, she also gave me a huge amount of freedom. As a teenager, I didn't appreciate it; my thoughts were more focused on grumbling about how "you never let me do anything." Now, when I look back, I think about what it would be like if I had kids, I doubt I would be able to give my kids the sort of freedom and support that my mum gave me.

As a kid, you just don't appreciate your parents. I don't tell my mum often enough about how incredibly grateful I am for the way she raised me. She had such a hard job. Like I said, my father disappeared – just walked out with no warning. Plus, the area we lived in was very rough. I know my mum has been subject to criticism from the rest of the family, but she just got on with it. In some ways, my mum served as a bit of a lesson, as to what not to do. She's inspired me not to make the same mistakes she made. So, yeah, my mum is my inspiration.

Like I mentioned, some of my motivation also comes from aging. I find myself getting more motivated as I get older. I see my mum aging. She recently turned 76. She's fine, just a few aches and pains. She still lives in the house where I grew up. As I watch her aging, I notice things changing. Once a practical, confident woman who easily made decisions, I see shades of doubt. I notice her confidence waning as she struggles to make decisions. I know this is a natural part of aging. I don't want that to happen to me. I want to keep pushing myself to try to stay as fit as I can.

Nowadays, you see so many people going out and doing things at amazing ages. I remember hearing about a woman recently who completed an Ironman at the age of 80-something. It's people like this that make you realize that age is just a number. I also think about people who were 60 in my nana's time. They were old. They acted old. They looked old. Today's 60-year-olds are aging differently. They are active. Healthy. Strong. In my running club, we have 60- and 70-year-olds who still run with the best of us.

In fact, there's a chap who likes to run 5Ks. He's 72. Almost 30 years his junior and I couldn't keep up with him. That's what motivates me: people like that who may not be as fast as they used to be, but they're still going out there and doing it.

I also think it's important to keep your body and your mind active. Obviously in life challenges come up. However, if you keep your mind and body strong, I think you have a better chance of overcoming those challenges.

Talking about motivation, I also think things like the *Tough Girl Podcast* are so important, especially for women. The media is full of rufty-tufty blokes doing things. I really don't see much coverage about what women are achieving. A couple of years ago, I went to the very first women's expedition expo in Bristol – I had no idea that there were so many women doing all these incredible things. Women just don't get the same exposure. That expo was incredibly motivating.

Hopefully that's [the negativity] changing a bit. In the UK, there has been a backlash about the lack of coverage of women's sports like women's football (soccer) and women's rugby. Unless you're a superstar trailblazer, female athletes just don't get the same media coverage. When you don't see people like you doing sports and getting into the outdoors, it's easy to overlook, not consider, or even discount that the possibility is even an option. Podcasts like *Sarah's Tough Girl Challenge* are an excellent way to hear about ordinary women doing incredible things. After listening, it's easy to think to yourself, "Well, they've done that, so why couldn't I?"

As you reflect on your accomplishments, what are one or two things that stand out the most for you?
Without a doubt, my 2016 Cho Oyu climb.

If you were to coach a friend, in a similar age range, who was thinking about trying a new sport or wanted to get out there to start moving, what would you tell them?

Take baby steps. The thing I find difficult, when I talk about what I've done all in one breath, it sounds like I'm some sort of super-human; I've done this, I've done that. It seems like there's not much I haven't done. This really isn't true. I want people to understand that I'm nothing special. I wasn't sporty at school, and I wasn't outdoorsy as a child. I just did little things here and there, bit by bit, building up my fitness. After trying something for the first couple of times, pretty soon I was thinking, "You know, I really enjoyed that." Then I did a bit more and thought, "Yeah, quite enjoyed that, too." Then, for me, the element of competition kicks in. I'll think, "Well, I can't really do that because that's an easier trek than the one I did before. I'm going to try this [harder] one."

If you were thinking of doing a trek somewhere, say Morocco, I would suggest starting out with a commercial company. Find a reputable company, take a look at their website, see what you fancy doing, and go from there. If you've got the money, the time, and the desire, sometimes the hardest thing is just hitting that submit button.

If somebody wanted to get into mountaineering, I would recommend some mountaineering courses as a good starting point. When I climbed Mount Ararat, that was my first experience with wearing crampons. They were the strap-on ones, the kind that strapped to your walking boots. I hadn't walked on crampons before, and we did a bit of crampon work before the climb. Then on Mera Peak, we were taught how to use a jumar, a fixed line, and things like that. But in all honesty, I had no idea what I was doing. Like I said, I was lucky.

In your mountaineering course, make sure you learn how to use an ice axe. If you slip and fall, it's really handy to know how to stop yourself. Using an ice axe is not easy or intuitive like you see in the movies. Plus, in the movies, they never, ever stop themselves or use an ice axe the right way.

Another important thing you might consider when climbing something like Mera Peak is safety. What if you find yourself in a position where the weather has turned, or your guide gets sick or falls and injures themselves? It's important to have the knowledge and skills so you can help keep things as safe as possible. I'm a big believer in making sure you get the tuition and skills you need before you head up any mountain.

I would also suggest that people join local clubs. I found a great mountaineering club near me. Joining this club gave me a chance to meet people who have the same interests and climb with people who are more experienced than me. You can see what they are doing, you can ask questions, which helps you learn. A club also gives you a safety net of other, more experienced people, to make sure you're not doing anything stupid. I've often done something completely daft. I just laugh and think to myself, "What was I thinking?" I find that sort of thing helps build confidence. I also joined a running club. I'm not the most social person, but through the clubs, I have met some really nice people. Plus, I have improved my running and trekking skills. Honestly, through trips, clubs, and courses, you'll soon find yourself connected to a community of like-minded people with similar interests.

I am fortunate that my job – as a civil servant – is quite flexible in a way that other industries might not be. For instance, they allowed me to take two months off work to climb Cho Oyu. I also don't have any ties. No children, no partner. So, I can please myself as to what I do and when I do it. If I had children, that might be different.

Money-wise, I don't earn a huge wage, but I also don't have an extravagant lifestyle; I plan and save for these trips. The Cho Oyu expedition was not cheap. To give you an idea, it took me 18 months to pay for it. In fact, for those 18 months, I was paying more per month for that trip than I was paying for my mortgage. I share this because I want people to know this kind of thing is within reach.

I can't stress enough the power of taking very small steps and allowing those steps to lead you to wherever it leads you. In my case, it led me to summit an 8,000-meter peak. Again, I really want people to know that I'm not special in anyway whatsoever. Honestly, I've got as many weaknesses, bad habits, and foibles as the next person. Believe me, if I can do it, you can do it.

If you had the one piece of sage advice to share with the world what would it be?

I think the main thing I want to say is don't put things off. You really don't know what's around the corner. It's easy to find every excuse not to do something: "I'm not ready," "This is a bad time," "I'm too old." We all get those thoughts.

If you've got your heart set on something and you're thinking, I would really like to do whatever it is, tell yourself, "Right, I'm going to do this, and this is when I'm going to do it." I know people can't always do things at the drop of a hat, but if you set yourself a time limit, make a plan, and tell yourself, "Right, I'm going to do this," then you'll get there.

Any final thoughts or reflections?

Believe me, I don't always follow my own advice because life does get in the way. It can be difficult to think about what you really want to do with your life. Please, if you get an opportunity to do something, you owe it to yourself to do it.

———

RICHARD 'BUTCH' BRITTON

Butch started running at 53. He's now 63. In the last six years,
Butch has completed 62 ultra-marathons, two 100-milers,
six or more 100-kilometer races and a dozen 50-milers.

*"I can wither away and become an old man, or
I can do something about it."*

– 'Butch' Britton

UNLIKE MY CONVERSATIONS with other athletes, Butch and Annie found me... That might sound strange; let me explain. My initial process started out with a Google search, a lead from a friend, or personal encounter. The first five interviews were very intentionally based on my personal interest, their coolness factor, like, "Wow! That's incredible. I want to be like that when I grow up," what they were accomplishing as athletes, or their age. Once identified, I reached out to the person directly in the hope that they would be willing to grant me an interview.

For Richard, better known as 'Butch', and Annie, who you will meet later – I used a different tactic. I did a 'wanted' post in a couple of running groups I belong to on Facebook. Butch and Annie responded. The universe outshined herself; there could not have been two more perfect people for the project. Butch's story is about pure grit and determination and captures the deep sense of community that lies at the heart of the trail and ultra-running communities.

I found Butch to be a funny, practical, straight-to-the-point kind of guy. Butch has a giving heart. He's served his country. Now, Butch serves his community which includes the families of veterans who have lost a loved one due to complexities of post-traumatic stress disorder (PTSD) and suicide. My conversation with Butch left me feeling grateful, humble, and inspired to keep moving into my 60s and beyond. Thank you, Butch!

Butch B

What is your favorite quote or saying?

The one that comes to my mind is from the movie *Cool Hand Luke* by Strother Martin: "What we have here is a failure to communicate." This quote helps remind me that, in life, you've got to be a good listener. That's my all-time favorite line.

Can you think of a book that stands out in your mind as an influential 'must read'?

Born to Run. Without a doubt. I started running when I was coaching high school baseball. One of the kids who played on the team was also on the cross-country team. The kid said, "Coach, you gotta read this book." So, I read the book. Honestly, it was that book that kicked off what I do now.

Please share a bit about your background. How did you get interested in this sport, and what were some of your first steps?

As a kid growing up, I was very, very competitive. I always wanted to win. Anything we were playing, whether it be cards, or board games, or sports, it was all about winning. I played baseball and wrestled. I wrestled throughout high school, college, and in the Marine Corps. Like I said, I was extremely competitive.

After high school, I tried college for a semester. I quickly realized college wasn't for me, so I dropped out and joined the Marine Corps. I was with them from 1973 to 1977. I wrestled for a short stint in the Marine Corps. I also played on the Quantico-based softball team. As a team, we traveled and played all over the East Coast. After I got out of the Marine Corps, I continued playing competitive softball. I traveled all over the United States playing in all kinds of tournaments. I continued playing well into my early 40s. I was in love with softball.

When I met my current wife, she had two children ages seven and eleven. Of course, her son was into baseball. So, I started coaching little league. Then her daughter wanted to play softball, so I coached a year of varsity fast-pitch softball. Coaching her team led to me coaching varsity baseball for the next 11 years.

As I look back, it was during this time that something began to shift. At this point in my life, I was 53 years old, working the daily grind at a bank. I remember one winter; I was staying at a lodge up on a lake in Minnesota. I was attending a national sales meeting for the bank. I was sitting next to this guy who looked amazing. He was all tan and looked very fit. Remember, this was in the depth of the Minnesota winter.

I knew this guy was from California. So, I asked him, "How come you're so tan?" He told me that he just got back from Kona. Intrigued, I asked, "What were you doing in Kona?" He elaborated, "Oh, the Ironman." I asked him how old he was. He said, "I'm 66." Not thinking I heard him correctly, I repeated, "You just did an Ironman?" "Yeah," he said, like it was no big deal.

The conversation with this guy hit me like a ton of bricks. I hadn't done anything exercise-wise for many, many years. The last time I did any serious running was in the Marine Corps almost 30 years ago.

I went home and took a long hard look in the mirror. I was 56 years old. I had a gut. I thought about my life. I went to work every day. I'd come home and give my wife a kiss on the cheek. I looked over at the couch and saw a big indentation from where my butt sat because I watched TV all the time. I told myself, "I've got to do something about this." It was at that moment when I realized I had a choice to make. I can wither away and become an old man, or I can do something about it. So, that very next day I got up, laced up, and ran a mile.

It nearly killed me. I ran one mile and felt like I was going to die. The next day I said, "OK, I'll go a mile and a quarter." And that killed me. Every day, running just kept on killing me. Just to give you an idea, it took me three months to get up to three miles.

I decided to enter a race. I entered the Marine Corps Marathon and signed up for the 10K distance. The race was in November. I registered for the race on July 5. I figured I could build my way up to a 10K in eight months.

So here I am, I'd run three miles. Pretty soon I was running four miles and slowly making my way up to five miles. At about the same time, my niece who is an officer in the Coast Guard asked if I wanted to enter a half marathon (13.1 miles) with her. Obviously, I had my doubts about whether I could do that distance. My niece said, no worries, "We'll run it together." So, I agreed. My niece and I ran the half marathon together. It killed me.

Also, around this time, I heard about the book *Born to Run*. I was fascinated by the stories about people running such incredible distances. It was funny because I had lived in Colorado for 13 years. I remember reading a story in the paper about these Indians running the Leadville 100-mile ultra-trail race. I honestly had no idea that all sorts of people across the world were running these kinds of races. I thought it was something fluky that was unique to this Indian tribe.

I did a bit of research and realized that the Leadville 100 was a legend. The Leadville 100 was *the* race that introduced the Tarahumara from Mexico's Sierra Madre mountains to the United States. Somewhere in all of this, I knew in my heart and soul I was determined to run an ultra-marathon.

Obviously, I had a long way to go. I slowly started to build up my mileage. I already had a half marathon under my belt. The next logical step was to sign up for a full marathon (26.2 miles).

I had no idea what I was doing. I read everything the internet had to offer about running. Back then, I didn't know a lot of runners, so I just gathered as much information as I could from articles and blogs and figured out what worked and what didn't. Eventually, I found a training plan I liked. Anyway, the following May, I ran my first marathon. It was hard, really hard, but I got it done.

I was ready for my first 50K. In June that same year, I signed up for my first ultra-marathon, the Dahlgren Heritage Trail 50K.

Man, I remember that summer. Every time I was

scheduled to do a long training run – say I was supposed to run 18 miles – it would be 100 degrees outside, and I'd manage 16 miles. The day I was supposed to run 20 miles, it would be even hotter outside; I would get 18 miles in and quit. It was like that all summer. I remember feeling so depressed about my training. I felt hopeless. I was constantly thinking to myself, "I am never going to be able to do this 50K."

I had to do something to get my head turned around, so I decided to run a local 25K trail race two weeks before the 50K. I looked at it like a training run to see how I did. Plus, I thought it might help build my confidence.

During the race, I met a father and son team. The dad, Mike, had been running ultra-marathons since the '90s. The duo was a good fit for my pace. I ended up running the race with them. The whole time I just grilled them for information. I had no running buddies, let alone a running community.

Those poor guys. I just peppered them with questions. "How do you do this?" "Why do you do that?" I was honest. I told them about my doubts and my fears about not physically being able to run that kind of distance. I remember leveling with Mike; "I just don't think I can do this." Mike said, "Look, just go down and start the race. The worst thing that can happen is you don't finish the race." I remember thinking to myself, "Yeah, I can do that."

Now my brain's like, "OK, I'll give it a shot." The 50K race was on my calendar for Sunday. That Friday night, justifying that I would be fine because I had until Sunday, I went to a party with some friends and drank excessively. I recall crashing sometime on Saturday morning. My next conscious memory is waking up to use the bathroom. As I walked past my office, I turned on the computer and I noticed the time – my race was in two hours! Plus, I had a two-hour drive. I had nothing packed. I started throwing stuff into a bag and flew out the door. I got to the race, missing the start by about 20 minutes. I registered, pinned on my bib, and filled up my water bottle. I said to myself, "Here we go. My first 50K..."

That day, the temperature climbed to over 100 degrees. I paired up with two guys who seemed to be going about the same pace. I literally ran with them and copied everything they did. At mile 20, one of the guys' support crew had ice-cold watermelon. I happen to love watermelon. I was thinking, "Oh, that sounds really good."

I made it to mile 20. Had some watermelon and started on the 11 miles back. By that time, the heat was horrendous, people were dropping like flies. I got about five miles out from the finish, when my running buddy said, "You got this. You can walk from here and still make it." I was like, "Wow, I have got this."

I did make it to the finish line. I completed my first ultra-marathon. I've got the hat to prove it! In the last six years, I've completed 62 ultra-marathons. I've done two 100-milers, six or so 100Ks, and maybe a dozen 50-milers.

Tell me about some of the joys, challenges, and milestones along the way.

Joys and challenges? I trained hard for my second 50K. That second 50K was my best ever. I felt so accomplished after that race, I decided to try and attempt one race a month. Out of the blue, I started to have issues with throwing up. At around mile 20, I'd just start puking. It took me almost 10 ultras to figure out what I should be eating and drinking. Figuring out the food/hydration thing was a big learning curve. I kept on doing 50Ks, and they kept on hurting really bad. I was beginning to wonder, "How am I ever going to do 50 miles? Nineteen more miles!" I just couldn't wrap my head around how to go from 31 to 50 miles.

After playing with that concept over and over in my brain for several years, I finally got the courage to enter a 50-mile race. It was great; went off without a hitch. I looked back and asked myself, "Why had I been stressing about this for so long?"

Thinking about food as fuel, what have you tried diet-wise? What has been helpful? Are there any supplements you swear by? Do you have any must-have foods when training or competing? What is a treat in your world?

I take some supplements: vitamins D, C, B12, iron, magnesium, potassium, fish oil, and glucosamine. I swear by glucosamine for my joints. I've had zero joint issues whatsoever.

When I'm training hard or racing, I use Tailwind. I put two scoops in a 20-ounce bottle. That's enough to give me about 200 calories per hour. Tailwind has all the electrolytes I need. Some people say you can race exclusively with just Tailwind. In a 100-mile race, I find my stomach saying, "Yeah, well it might have all the calories I need, but I'm hungry." So, I also eat solid food. Now I'm over that puking thing, I can eat most anything. I like peanut butter sandwiches. I love pizza. I like hamburgers. Peanut M&Ms, chips, you name it! When I'm at the aid station, I just grab a handful of stuff and keep on moving. After a race, my all-time favorite treats are watermelon and orange slices.

How did you begin to build your fitness? What were some of your early steps? And how did you know you were starting to form a habit?

When I looked in the mirror after that conference in Minnesota, I knew I had to make some major changes. I think I was literally scared into getting those running shoes on and heading out the door.

In the beginning running was brutal. I started small; first a mile. Then a mile and a quarter. It took at least three months of slowly adding distance for my body to begin to adjust to running. Somewhere along the way I read *Born to Run*. At that point, I just knew deep in my heart I wanted to run ultra-marathons.

Do you have any morning or evening routines?

I like to run in the evening. It relieves the stress from the day. However, when I do my long runs on the weekends, I like to get out early in the morning.

Discrimination and/or negativity as an older athlete – do you think this is a thing? Have you personally experienced it? How did you deal with it? What would you tell others?

Actually, my experience has been exactly the opposite. The trail and ultra-running community are a very close-knit group of people. From my very first race, I met some people. I went to more races and met more people. The more races you do, the more people you meet. Because you are running such long distances, you often end up running with people for hours. Plus, the ultra-community is pretty small, so you keep running – no pun intended – into the same people again and again.

When I first started running, I joined some trail running groups. I'm a pretty social person. I'd show up at an event, notice someone wearing a T-shirt from one of the groups I belonged to, and go up and introduce myself, "Hey, I'm from so and so." Pretty soon we're striking up a conversation – I have met so many amazing people along the way.

There are guys older than me running. Because I started much later in life, I am one of the older, less experienced runners. Some of the old-timers have been running since the '80s. They're career runners. Because I'm one of the older guys, I get asked a lot of questions. People want my advice. As a later-in-life athlete, I have been welcomed and respected. I have experienced no sense of discrimination. I have felt accepted and valued, more like a mentor.

We all have thoughts that can be negative: fears, doubts, that critical voice that might say, "Who do you think you are?" or "What are you thinking? You can't do that." What are some tips and tricks you use to combat your own 'stinking thinking'?

That's a great question... Previously I mentioned getting sick and throwing up during my early races. I remember feeling so bad during those races, in my head I would promise myself, "Never again." I would tell myself, "I am never going to do this again, ever. This is my last race. I've had it. I can't do this anymore." Then another little voice would start, "Look, you've only got two miles to the next aid station, you can do this." I'd be hating life, kicking, and screaming but somehow I'd make it to the next aid station. I'd drink some ginger ale or some Coke. I'd have something to eat, then my mind was like, "OK, you've only got five miles left. You can do that."

Factors like this have shaped the way I run races today. It's because of these rookie situations that I learned to use an aid-station-to-aid-station strategy. I have learned to not think about time. I don't think about my pace. I don't think about anything. My thoughts are 100% focused on getting to the next aid station. For instance, when you're running a 100-miler, it's a given that at some point you're going to feel like your legs are shot. When I get to that point, I personally don't like walking the rest of the way; that takes forever. So, I make a deal with myself. I'll tell myself, "OK, run to that tree up ahead, then you can walk for a bit." Between the aid stations and points along the trail, I break down the 100 miles into smaller, more manageable steps. That's how I get though the negativity.

As for failures, sure, I've had failures. I remember when I stepped up to the 100s. I had run a 50-miler in November. I felt I was ready for my first 100. I signed up for the C&O Canal 100. The race was the following April. Remember, this was early on in my running career; I still didn't know much about ultra-running.

Anyway, I got to mile 40 and started to notice pain in my heels. I had never had any problems with my feet, so I was kind of surprised. I stopped at the next aid station and picked up my drop bag. I took off my shoes and socks and saw two massive blisters, one on each heel.

The guy sitting next to me looks over and offers to fix the blisters for me. I said, "Sure." Going into the aid station, my discomfort level was about a two on a one-to-10 scale – 10 being searing pain. So, the guy proceeds to pop and tape my blisters. Instantly, the level of pain level skyrockets to an 11. I switched out shoes, thinking that would help. I couldn't walk a step. I tried another pair of shoes. I still couldn't walk. The pain was so bad I literally could not take another step. I couldn't walk. I couldn't run. At mile 40, I dropped out.

The following year, I signed up for the C&O Canal 100 again. This time I got to mile 40 when it started to pour with rain. I knew when I got to mile 50 I would be able to get my rain jacket from my drop bag. At that point, the daytime temperature was in the 50s. Over the next hour or so, we had four inches of rain and temperatures falling into the mid-30s.

I got to mile 60. This was the turn-around point, and the aid station where I had planned to meet my pacer. I remember the race director and his girlfriend checking in on me. "Hey, Butch, how are you doing?" they asked. They gave me a strange look and inquired again. "Hey, Butch, how are you doing?" By that time, I had all the symptoms of hyperthermia, which included the inability to talk. They pulled me from the race. Another failed attempt.

The following spring, I finally completed my first 100-miler, the Umstead 100. I continued to struggle with blisters. This time, blisters or no blisters, I was determined to earn my buckle. I had blisters so big they covered the balls on the bottom of both feet. Regardless, I still finished and have my first buckle to prove it. I was overjoyed!

I could not shake the C&O 100-miler, so I decided to tackle it again. Third time's a charm. The race was in April. The weather served up a sweltering 95 degrees. By mile 53, I was overheated and throwing my guts up. I had blisters on both feet and my quads were seizing up. It was bad. I dropped out at mile 53. Now, I'm zero for three at the C&O 100.

Over time, I have learned to work with my body and my mind. There's nothing I can do about hypothermia. I can deal with blisters and I can deal with throwing up. Believe me, I've had to learn how to deal with plenty of negative thoughts rushing though my head: "I hate this. This sucks!" "Never again!" Now, I can push through the negativity by using positive thoughts and bargaining with myself to get me to that next aid station. Honestly, that's how I run my races: one aid station at a time. This year I went back to the C&O 100 – my fourth attempt. I finally got that buckle. And, I managed to beat my best 100-mile time by two hours.

Injuries & illness – have you had any major setbacks health-wise? How do you cope with injuries? Do you do anything to avoid injuries? What tips do you have for healing and recovery?

Right after my first half marathon, I got plantar fasciitis (PF). The podiatrist suggested insoles. So, I got insoles. Then she referred me to a physical therapist. The physical therapist was great. He asked me if I wanted to learn how to treat the PF myself. I quickly replied, "Oh yes!" He taught me all the stretches, all the rolls, all the things you're supposed to do. Now and again, I'll get a flare-up; overall, it hasn't been a problem.

This year, for some reason, I had a flare-up three weeks before my 100-miler. The PF came back hard. For three days, I used all the tools my PT taught me. By day four, I was fine. I made it through 100 miles, no problem.

I'd love to hear about what inspires you… Who are your role models? How do you stay motivated?

I am a veteran. Things that adversely affect veterans and their families are close to my heart. The first 100-miler I ran, I dedicated to the Wounded Warrior Project. The race was also a fundraiser. Although I didn't finish the race, I did raise close to $1,500. It felt good to use running to raise money and awareness to help veterans returning home from war.

As I started to dig into the Wounded Warrior Project a bit more, I wasn't happy with what I was finding. Frankly, I was disgruntled about the percentage of money going to veterans versus what the organization was keeping. This really got my goat.

About two years ago, I ran into this group called '22 Too Many' a nonprofit organization that supports our military communities, their families, and their loved ones to deal with grief, loss, suicides, and PTSD. To give you some perspective, since 1990, about 8,000 people have been killed in the Middle East. Over the same time period, almost 200,000 veterans have committed suicide. According to the U.S. Department of Veterans Affairs, every day, 22 veterans take their own lives.

Being former military myself, I felt compelled to do something. I became a supporter of 22 Too Many. I started running for the cause. It's simple. Go to the organization's home page and select someone from the 'Heroes' page. 22 Too Many provides the hero's name, his or her picture, and some background information about the veteran. You show up on race day with the picture of the person on your back. Your run is dedicated to the veteran who has died by suicide. Photos are taken and shared, honoring the veteran and increasing awareness.

I started running races with a picture of a veteran who has died by suicide pinned to the back of my shirt. During the race, people ask about what I am doing. I talk about the person I am running for and tell them about 22 Too Many. At this point, I have run for more than 20 veterans.

I have actually taken this a bit further. Whenever I get a finisher's prize, I send the prize, along with a personal letter, to the parents, wife, or child of the veteran who had committed suicide. I've received five or six letters in return telling me how uplifting it is to know that somebody's thinking about the loved one they have lost.

This issue has also hit really close to home. Last year, my best friend in the Marine Corps lost his son to PTSD. His boy committed suicide. When I found out, I told my friend about my mission to bring awareness to PTSD. With his picture on my back, I ran the C&O Canal 100 in his son's honor. His surviving son, an officer in the Navy, and his daughter showed up at around mile 40 to support me. As you can imagine, that was a powerful moment. Getting involved and feeling like I am doing something that makes a difference – that's my motivation.

As you reflect on your accomplishments, what are one or two things that stand out the most for you?

Any ultra-runner will tell you that the ultimate goal is to receive the 100-mile buckle – the prized belt buckle awarded to finishers of a 100 mile-race. For me, receiving my first buckle at the Umstead 100 in North Carolina felt like a huge accomplishment. There's nothing like the feeling of winning that first buckle.

If you were to coach a friend, in a similar age range, who was thinking about trying a new sport or wanted to get out there to start moving, what would you tell them?

I would want to remind people of two things: one, for any new activity, it takes 21 days for our muscle memory system to kick in, and two, start slow. Walk if you can't run. If you are morbidly obese or horribly out-of-shape, begin with a 10-minute walk to the mailbox and back. Start small. Start somewhere. Pretty soon, your legs will get used to walking. Once you build stamina with walking, try running for a couple of seconds. Then begin to alternate walking with a couple of minutes of running. Of course, I didn't take my own advice. When I first started out, I remember running that first mile and feeling like I was going to die. Not a good idea.

Over time, you will get stronger. Also, don't worry about your time or speed. So many people are worried about running that six-minute mile, or a sub – fill in the blank – 5K or 10K. That's often the mentality of people who run on roads. Like I said earlier, I am super competitive by nature, but I have learned to put that part of me aside. If you can carry on a conversation while you're running, then you're running at the right speed. If you're huffing and puffing, gasping for air, and speaking in one-word sentences, then you're going too fast. Remember, time does not matter. What does matter is getting out there and moving.

I've used a run/walk method in my training for longer distance races. I remember one spring when I was struggling with plantar fasciitis and got sick with the flu – I just couldn't run. So, I walked. I did a 20-mile walk. Then I did another 20-mile walk. Then I did a 31-mile walk. I completed that 100-miler using a cycle of 40 seconds of running with two minutes of walking. It took me 26 and a half hours to complete the race. Honestly, that was the easiest 100-mile race I ever completed. I had absolutely no problems throughout the entire race. Now, I'm training for another 100-miler using the same method. I did a 20-mile walk last week. I have another one scheduled in a couple weeks. For me it's all about completion. I just want to finish the race.

It's also about having fun. The ultra-running community is very supportive and social. I enjoy the post-race atmosphere, when runners are hanging out enjoying their favorite adult beverage, just sitting around and chatting – I love it! In short, here's my advice for people starting out: slow down, listen to your body, go out and find a running or walking buddy, have a conversation, and just enjoy the heck out of it.

If you had the one piece of sage advice to share with the world what would it be?

Life is all about giving back to the community. That's something I feel strongly about. For me, giving back has come in many ways, from coaching baseball to running for people who have lost their lives through suicide.

Look for opportunities to lend a hand. If you're in a race and you spot someone struggling, come alongside, support them, help them get to the finish line. There have been times when I have shut down my race to get someone through to the finish. Remember to give back.

Any final thoughts or reflections?

Please stay active. As we age and move toward retirement, it's vital to keep moving. At least get out and walk. After all, what good is it to work your entire life then get to retirement and get struck with some debilitating disease and die?

Whether it's riding a bike, using an elliptical, or getting out and walking; find something you enjoy and do it regularly – it's so important! Don't take my word for it, there is a mountain of evidence supporting the benefits of regular movement including lower cholesterol, lower blood pressure and glucose levels, which means less heart disease and conditions like diabetes.

Exercise is also a great stress reliever. Let's face it, we can all use that. My final advice for people is to take 30 minutes out of your day and exercise. Get outside. Go for a walk. Breathe in some fresh air and see what a difference it makes to the way you feel.

———

YVONNE ENTINGH
AKA PRINCESS DOAH
Solo Female Endurance Hiker

"Life is an adventure, life is a journey, and life is passion. Adventure, journey, and passion – to me that's life!"

– Yvonne Entingh

MY PATH CROSSED WITH YVONNE'S thanks to a Google search. I was looking for a backpacking course for beginners. Yvonne, the owner and fearless leader of her own small adventure company, happened to be offering a Backpacking 101 weekend. So, I signed up with absolutely no idea what to expect.

Although I am no stranger to the trail, with regard to this trip, I was a blank slate in two ways. First, I was completely new to backpacking, and second, the idea for this book project, or any book project for that matter was so far out of my consciousness I would have laughed, scoffed, or rolled my eyes at such a ridiculous notion, "Me, write a book, yeah, right!"

My goals for the backpacking weekend were simple: to learn how to pitch a tent, pack a backpack, and, of vital importance, figure out how the heck you pack enough food and snacks for three days.

As the weekend unfolded, I learned Yvonne, also known by her trail name Princess Doah, was a highly experienced backpacker with thousands and thousands of, mostly solo, miles under her belt. I had never met anyone, let alone a woman, with an outdoor résumé like Yvonne's. Yvonne, with her humble demeanor, and her quiet, yet powerful presence, was my new superhero. Sure, I had read about people (mostly men) through books, articles, and talks – but never up close and personal. I began to realize that Yvonne was, indeed, a unique human.

I vividly recall sitting around the campfire that first evening listening to Yvonne humbly share a little about her journey. Her memories as a child watching the men in her family prepare for trips in the backwoods and her excitement about hearing about their adventures upon their return. Yvonne also told us about the powerful influence Grandma Gatewood had on her hiking/backpacking adventures, as she spoke you could literally feel the deep sense of joy, passion, and deep connection Yvonne has to the outdoors.

During our conversation Yvonne tells us, very candidly, about some of her personal joys, fears, and challenges that go hand-in-hand with being out on the trail for months at a time. Woven in between

Yvonne's words I hope you will find another thread. An awareness. A deeper felt sense that conveys Yvonne's love for the natural world.

The brief time I've spent with Yvonne has influenced my life in two ways. My love for backpacking was ignited, and the seed for this book was planted. Sometimes it's a challenge to find the right words to describe deeper felt emotions. My hope is that this conversation inspires a spark of a curiosity about the wonders and healing nature of the natural world. Yvonne, I can't thank-you enough...

Yvonne E

What is your favorite quote or saying?

There are lots of quotes out there; this one has really stuck with me.

"Never, never, never give up..." by Winston Churchill.

I saw this quote in Key West when I was hiking the southern portion of the Eastern Continental Divide trail. I took a picture of it... Since then, I have used this quote literally thousands of times.

Can you think of a book that stands out in your mind as an influential 'must read'?

The Bible. Definitely the Bible...

Please share a bit about your background. How did you get interested in this sport, and what were some of your first steps?

This is a question a lot of people ask me... I have always been outdoorsy. I always had a garden, even when I was little. I loved playing in the dirt and just loved being outside. I think I was strongly influenced by having parents who got us outdoors. As a kid, every Sunday after church, we'd go on a family picnic or have a cookout. We'd go hiking. We'd be outdoors somewhere. I remember us taking off in the car, not knowing where we would end up. We'd stop along a county road. We'd take a walk in the field or along a stream. We would always have an adventure somewhere.

We also took vacations every year. Our vacations were nothing elaborate. We would pack the car and head off to the Smokey Mountains or Michigan. We basically spent a week or so outside, camping, swimming, hiking, and playing out in nature.

As a kid I was also influenced by my father and brother. Throughout the years, my father and brother would get together with our cousins and uncles. A group of them, always just the men, would head off to Canada. I remember watching them prepare for their trips. They planned, talked about food, and packed their gear which included canoes and backpacking equipment. When it came time for us to say our goodbyes as they headed off for their great adventure I remember, even as a little kid, feeling intrigued – I wanted to go too.

After, what seemed like weeks, they returned home. I remember listening, wide-eyed, to their wonderful stories about all their adventures. Stories about campfires and eating porridge, spotting moose, skinny-dipping, and drinking straight from crystal clear lakes and streams. Dad would always bring me home a small gift; a birch bark canoe or something made by an Indian. I just loved that...

What got me into backpacking, boy, I don't know? Suddenly, I had this interest and I thought I would explore it. I remember going to a local presentation hosted by the Five Rivers Metro Parks in Dayton, Ohio. I think it was called Backpacking Basics or something like that. They had a PowerPoint. They had backpacks. They went over all the gear and showed us what they took out with them.

Intrigued, I decided to sign up for an overnight backpacking trip. A group of us headed out. We walked to the location, set up our tents and camped. It was more like car camping. But it was enough to spark my interest. The same group happened to be hosting an Appalachian Trail (AT) hike. I wanted to sign up to for the AT hike. The hike was full; I put my name on the waiting list just in case.

The following year the organizers called me and said, "Hey, you were on a waiting list last year. Would you be interested in hiking the AT this year?"

I hesitated and explained, "I have never done anything like this before. I don't know if I can keep up. And I don't know what to take…" I instantly had all these questions and doubts flying through my head. I agreed to go. I also asked if my brother could go with me. He's been in the back country before. The man I was talking to happened to know my brother. He knew his abilities and agreed that he could come too. So, that was it!

We hiked 27 miles in the Shenandoah National Park on the Appalachian Trail. After that, I did two Red River Gorge trips and a trip to Shawnee with a group of people from a local hiking club. The following year, over the Memorial Day Weekend, I did my first solo hike – 30-something miles on the Appalachian Trail over three days. I was hooked!

I just love everything about it… I love the breeze in my hair and the feeling of the sun on my face. I love the wonder about what's around that next curve in the trail. I also like the physical hardship and the endurance aspect of backpacking. I love the challenge, mentally and physically.

For me, when I'm out there on the trail by myself, there's a sense of independence and a sense of freedom. I don't have to answer to anyone for anything. When I first started, some of my first realizations were how much I enjoyed making my own decisions and how much I enjoyed the challenge of not just surviving, but thriving. The choices I make for the day. The water sources. The food re-supply. The camping decisions. I have to figure all that out.

I'm a planner by nature, so I think that helps. Plus, I'm pretty organized – that's just part of my character. I honestly believe that God has given me these abilities to do the things I am doing today. It's difficult to describe… I literally yearn to be outside. I yearn to be in the mountains. I meditate. I pray.

This is the time where I connect with God. I depend on Him when I'm out there. Because of the distractions of everyday life and the responsibilities at home, I don't want to say all that keeps me from my faith, but when I'm out there, all day I feel this powerful energy and connection with Jesus Christ. Like I said, it's difficult to put into words.

Tell me about some of the joys, challenges, and milestones along the way.

Joys. Oh, boy. I have had so many joys. I remember when I first started backpacking, I was still working and had a limited schedule, so I section-hiked the Appalachian Trail. Every time I went out and had to leave the trail to head home, I cried. I felt so sad; just this incredible sense of loss. When I first started backpacking these feelings were difficult to handle. This sense of loss hasn't gone away. Recently, I hiked the Long Trail and cried at the end of the trail. Yes, I was tired. Yes, I was ready to rest; I was incredibly sad the journey was over.

There are very real challenges related to going back home after extended periods on the trail. The adjustment is hard. Once I'm home, I still eat trail food. I sleep on the floor. I wear the same clothes. I'm not ready to jump back into everyday life.

Another joy, oh my word, that would be the people I have met along the way. I don't think folks realize that there is a lot of road walking on many of the major trail systems. The Mountains-to-Sea trail has about 600 miles of road. The Florida Trail, the Alabama sections of the Eastern Continental Trail have hundreds of miles of road walking as does the American Discovery Trail. The Appalachian Trail is one of the exceptions.

The people I've met may not have been on the trail itself, but on the road sections. I can tell you story after story about the incredible things I have experienced. Everything from people reaching out and inviting me into their home. To people giving me shelter from the rain. To people doing my laundry or offering a kind word or giving me a bottle of water. I can't tell you how many times I have been walking along and someone drove by and reached their arm out the window with a bottle of fresh, cold water on a hot day. They don't say a word. They drive off and go on about their day.

A recent example of the extraordinary trail magic I received was while I was backpacking through Delaware, Maryland, and West Virginia on the Eastern Section of the American Discovery Trail. The American Discovery Trail is a collection of trails and roads that span 6,800 miles across America from the Atlantic Ocean to the Pacific Ocean. Unless you order an Uber, have a hotel reservation, and pizza delivery on speed dial, in many areas, there are limited opportunities to get off the trail and into town.

I hiked close to 500 miles of this trail during July and August. I know that hiking during the summer months has its own set of challenges. I am prepared for the long hot days, high humidity, and the bugs – this trip was no exception.

Local people, those familiar with the trail, would see me out there on the road with my backpack, and literally pull over and ask, "Hey, where are you spending the night?" They would explain that they live a few miles down the road, just off the trail. So many people offered me a place to stay, along with a chance to cool off and rehydrate. The experience of receiving so much kindness and generosity from complete strangers is one of the things I cherish.

As for challenges, I have sure had those as well. I remember when I first started out, I was naïve; there were so many things I hadn't considered. For instance, harsh weather. I'm not particularly fond of storms. When lightning and thunder are crashing right over my head, that's a real challenge for me. Over time, I have learned to keep calm and react in a flash of a moment. I usually take off my pack, quickly find shelter, and wait it out. Another challenge can be the terrain. The roughness of the trail. Having to resupply and then carry the extra weight of four or five days of food and water on my back can be a challenge.

There are also challenges related to being a solo female hiker. One that comes to mind are road crossings. Whether it be a forest-service road, a gravel road, or even a busy road. Before I get to a road, I want to be very aware. I want to know exactly which way the trail goes. While I'm in the woods, before I get to the road crossing, I take out my map, study it, and make sure I know exactly where I am going. I just don't think it's good practice for a woman to be pulling out her map when she gets to a road. It indicates, "I don't know what I'm doing, and I don't know where I am." If I'm way out there I make sure I know exactly what's around me – are there parked cars? Are they empty? Who's in the car? Is it a male? The same rules apply if I am hitch-hiking into town to resupply. I'm not sure that these are so much challenges; it's more about common sense and awareness.

Thinking about food as fuel, what have you tried diet-wise? What has been helpful? Are there any supplements you swear by? Do you have any must-have foods when training or competing? What is a treat in your world?

For the past several years my diet has been gluten and dairy free. I'm not paleo, but I'm grain-free to some extent. I'm not a big meat-eater. When I'm home my eating style is fairly simple. When I'm out on the trail, those food choices are still doable; it just takes a bit more planning. I'll usually ship out a resupply box to a local outfitter, post office, or trail town I'll be passing through.

I make a lot of my own food. My dehydrator is generally busy, humming along in the weeks leading up to a trip preparing meals. My family worries about me not getting enough protein when I'm out on the trail. When I'm out on the trail I'll eat chicken and turkey jerky. I used to eat tuna and salmon, but I've really cut back on all that. I choose grass fed organic products. I don't eat junk food. Recently, I have really cut back on my sugar intake. I make sure I am getting enough electrolytes and salty foods.

As for supplements, I take magnesium and a women's daily vitamin. I take goji berries and other herbs. I love herbal teas. I don't drink coffee or soda. Dark chocolate is probably my comfort food. It's interesting, I think I eat well at home. When I'm on the trail, I eat even better.

I used to be pretty strict about the food I packed for the trail. Food weighs a lot, especially when you're carrying enough food for five or six days. Nowadays, I don't worry about the weight so much. I eat whatever I want to eat out there. If I want fresh fruit, I'll take fresh fruit. I'll take things like avocados which will last two or three days. I make sure I have nuts. I love cashews.

My favorite comfort food is probably peanut butter. I love peanut butter. I take dried peanut butter and add water to it. Then, of course, there's chocolate. It's not an everyday thing, but yeah, I like to have dessert. At this point in my life my attitude is more laid back, if I have to carry it, then so be it...

How did you begin to build your fitness? What were some of your early steps? And how did you know you were starting to form a habit?

When I first started backpacking one of my fears was not being able to keep up with the group. I wanted to make sure I was in good shape, so I didn't slow people down. I remember training every day for my first backpacking trip. I trained like I was going to run a marathon. I forget what my exact routine looked like; I know I started out hiking a couple of days a week. Then, once I was comfortable, I started carrying a full pack on those hikes. As I got stronger, I gradually increased my distance to seven, then 10, then 12, until I was able to hike 14 miles comfortably with a full pack on my back.

As far as a routine, boy, I'm a trail runner. Well, I'm a trail trotter. I don't run or jog. I trot. I get out once or twice a week to run. I also do stairs. We have local parks in my area that have some great stairs. I also recommend yoga to athletes. Yoga is very important for strength, flexibility, coordination, and balance. I have a Meetup page where I post free yoga classes and invite others to join me.

Generally, my routine looks like this: Mondays – yoga; Tuesdays – run; the rest of the week I add mileage with hiking. Of course, sometimes things come up. Like this week for instance, I am completely off routine and haven't been outside once. I just make sure to get back on track quickly. During the winter I join a gym and take Total Resistance Exercise (TRX) classes. TRX is a form of suspension training that uses body weight exercises to develop strength, balance, and flexibility. I find this is a great way to build upper body strength which is important for backpacking. I also try to get out and hike as much as possible.

Do you have any morning or evening routines?

Each day starts at 7:30 am when I connect with my church for praise and worship time. My church has a huge community with people all over the world. We connect via Facebook. We sing. There is a Bible reading. We share comments and posts. I am a prayer warrior. I pray daily and throughout the day.

Every morning I wake up and say, "Good morning, Father. Good morning, Jesus. Good morning, Holy Spirit." I start praying while I'm in bed. Then at the close of the day I fall asleep praying. After I get up, I make my bed – I feel so much better when the house is clean and tidy. Then I eat. That's my routine!

Discrimination and/or negativity as an older athlete – do you think this is a thing? Have you personally experienced it? How did you deal with it? What would you tell others?

That's a good question. Quite honestly, I haven't experienced any discrimination. In fact, it's been the complete opposite. For sure, I get interest, surprise, and questions. I remember one section of the American Discovery Trail where I didn't see a soul for miles except for a stretch where, on three separate occasions, I saw young men hiking solo. As we stopped to chat, each one of them commented, "Wow, you're the first female I've seen out here backpacking." Often the conversation moves from surprise, to questions and concerns, "You're a woman out here alone... aren't you scared with everything that's going on in the world?" I get questions; as far as discrimination, feeling left out or and shamed – no, that has not been my experience. People have been supportive and interested; I have felt nothing but respect and admiration.

As for my family, I am the mother of three adult daughters. I am also a daughter and a grandmother. It's important to realize that this lifestyle was completely new to my family. It took them a while to come to terms with the fact that their mom was now a solo female endurance hiker. And that this was a *huge* part of my life.

I know my girls worry about me. They are concerned when I am gone for months at a time. They get nervous about me falling and injuring myself. They imagine me all alone, out in the backwoods. They fret about "all the dangers." They question my safety and want to know how I'm going to protect myself. Of course, I know that they love me and want me to be okay.

Despite their concerns, my family has been incredibly supportive. When I finished the Appalachian Trail, my family threw a 'congratulations' party for me. They were proud of my accomplishments and thought it was great. I had been home for three months, then I was off again, flying down to Key West to hike another 2,000 miles up to the Appalachian Trail. Once I had completed that trail, I started to plan my next adventure.

I know at times my choices have been difficult, or confusing, for my family to accept. I remember the day when one of my daughters expressed, "Mom, I have finally realized that I believe this is your ministry. This is where God has put you and this is your ministry." This was a turning point. Receiving my children's acceptance was huge.

Now we have an understanding. They want to know where I'm going and when I'll be back. They also want to know how to get ahold of me when I'm out on the trail. I leave them a detailed itinerary. I keep in touch as often as possible. I also carry a GPS tracking device. When I'm in an area with no cellular coverage I can send a brief update. Plus, I can signal emergency services if needed.

By being out on the trail, starting my business, doing presentations, and just talking to people, I believe this is God's way of giving me a platform. It just took a while for my family to get used to my new normal.

Again, as far as discrimination goes, for me it's been the opposite. I know I am well respected in the community because of the feedback I get. People see me getting older. They see me in good health and still getting out there – doing what I love to do. I find people applaud that. People are inspired.

We all have thoughts that can be negative: fears, doubts, that critical voice that might say, "Who do you think you are?" or "What are you thinking? You can't do that." What are some tips and tricks you use to combat your own 'stinking thinking'?

I remember doing a presentation hosted by Wright State University for the local Metro Parks system titled, '*Fear* Is Not an Option'. I talked about the fears I had and the 'what-if thinking'. As a society we have become so fearful of the 'what-ifs'. We clog-up our minds with unhelpful thoughts and negative thinking patterns. Pretty soon this style of thinking can become overwhelming, leading to worry, anxiety, and fear.

People often ask me if I am scared. Generally, my answer is simple, "...I have peace because I know who is in control. God is. I know that He's got my back. No matter what happens, He is going to be there with me."

As far as fears go, nobody I know likes to sleep outside, way out there, far away from anybody, in the dark. I tend to have more apprehensions than fears. My apprehensions generally center around bad weather, getting injured, and road crossings. Seeing lightning in the area or knowing I am coming up on a road crossing are definitely times when I feel a bit more anxious. Learning what to do when lightning is close by, knowing how to get off the trail if I'm injured, and being prepared for road crossings help me stay calm.

I also rely on that sixth sense they say we all have. Be aware. If you sense that someone is being a creeper or has bad intentions – listen to that. Being aware of your surroundings is *vital*. Boy, I can't stress that enough...

Recently, I was down in Florida for five weeks with my mom. I wanted to do some of the Florida Trail, so I did Ocala. I forget how many miles it is... Anyway, I took off out on the trail. There's a section of the Ocala trail that takes you through the Juniper

Springs Wilderness. I didn't know this, but apparently there had been some bear activity in the area. Bears don't bother me. If they're out there, they're out there. In my mind, they don't bother me. In southern Florida, they also have panthers; that's another story.

So, I'm on the trail, up north, above Orlando when I sensed something in my gut. It was just a feeling; a sense. I stopped. I turned around and looked. I wasn't speaking out loud, or singing, or anything. I had to have stopped and looked around me at least five times. I would take a few steps; get this sense; and stop and look around. I looked up in the trees and looked around on the ground. Nothing.

I wasn't overcome by fear. I just kept sensing something. The sixth time I stopped, turned around, and looked I just stood very still for a moment. When I turned back around to face the trail, something on the left side of me, hidden deep among the Saw Palmetto and dense under-brush, growled. Some-thing growled real low.

I'm thinking, "OK, bears don't growl." I quickly realized it could be a panther. My first reaction was to pull the straps on my backpack up higher so that my neck was covered. This is a tip: when you're out there in wildlife, know which part of your body an animal might attack. Panthers and mountain lions generally go for the head and the back of the neck.

I quickly pulled my pack up as high as possible so that it was higher than my head and started walking. No more stopping. No more looking around. Then I immediately started quoting scripture, out loud, talking; talking to God. I was literally praying out loud, "Father, even the winds and the seas obey you. You created this animal," or however I worded it, "and he is under your command and your control." I just kept walking and praying; walking and praying.

I finally reached a road crossing. I was happy to see a local hunter/tracker who happened to be passing through. He stopped long enough to have a conversation about the wildlife in the area. As a tracker and a hunter, he hadn't seen any evidence of large cats. Later I met up with some nomadic hikers. Nomadic hikers are people that stay out in the backwoods for months on end. They were very familiar with that area. As we were talking, they confirmed evidence of large cat activity, "Oh, yeah," they said. "We've seen them and their prints out here."

Experiencing the power of that sixth sense was the weirdest feeling. I'm just walking along quite happily, then out of nowhere – something inside me warns me to be hyper aware. To continuously turn around, looking, and listening. I'm not 100% sure it was a panther. However, when I googled the sound, that low growl – it was definitely something.

Again, I can't express how important it is to be aware of your surroundings. To develop and use that sixth sense. Know what to do in a situation when you're confronted with something like that. I wasn't fearful. I wasn't anxious. I knew I had to react. I quickly pulled my pack up and put one of my trekking poles behind my legs. I had to protect my neck and my legs. Not that this would have done much if I was attacked. Regardless, I was ready and prepared. Panthers and mountain lions are out there. Just like house cats, they stalk their prey.

Injuries & illness – have you had any major setbacks health-wise? How do you cope with injuries? Do you do anything to avoid injuries? What tips do you have for healing and recovery?

Yes, I've had injuries and illnesses for sure! I got norovirus when I was on the AT and had to take a day off. I have fallen on the trail many times. Last year, when I was hiking the New England National Scenic Trail, I did a complete face plant. I literally slid my face into the ground. To make matters worse, I had my glasses on. The glasses smashed into my face injuring my nose and eyes. I chipped a tooth. It felt like my teeth were rattling in my head. I managed to scrape myself up and sat and rested for a while. I hiked the next day. Then I took a zero day. I wasn't doing well. My head was really hurting. Eventually, common sense kicked in; I decided to go home and get checked out.

I made it home and went to the doctor. I had a

bad concussion. I got my teeth looked at. That fall took me off the trail for the rest of the year. I hate that feeling of not finishing what I set out to accomplish.

I remember another time on the Mountains-to-Sea trail, about 800 miles into the hike, my left lliotibial band (IT) band and knee area would not quit hurting. I would literally take a few steps then have to stop and rest. I knew I needed to get it looked at. So, I got off the trail and found a doctor. They did some X-rays, gave me a cortisone shot, some medication, and direct orders, "to rest." I did go home and rest, then, once I got the all clear, went back out there and finished that trail. Although it did not end up being a through hike, I did finish the Mountains-to-Sea trail in about eight months.

Since then my knees do tend to hurt. When I'm out on the trail. I wear knee braces. I also have bursitis in my right shoulder. Yoga helps that tremendously. I have also struggled with chronic blisters, to the point where my feet just bleed. So, I also take really good care of my feet. I have learned that doing too much too soon can cause a lot of these problems.

Believe me, making the decision to get off the trail is hard. I feel disappointment along with a sense that I have let myself down by not meeting the expectations I set for myself. Over time, I have had to learn that I'm not a failure. I may not have accomplished what I set out to do, but *I'm* not a failure. I've learned to put aside my thoughts about what 'other people might think'.

I know I tend to push myself. Another thing I've learned is how important it is to listen to your body. After those two injuries, I knew the best thing, in the long run, was to come home to rest and recover.

I'd love to hear about what inspires you... Who are your role models? How do you stay motivated?

How do I stay motivated? Wow! Mentally, I think I have a good mental disposition, I'm not sure that's the right word? People say that to be a solo hiker, you must be comfortable with yourself. You're by yourself all day every day. You're constantly thinking and planning. That's what I do. I think, I plan, and I execute things in my mind.

I think it's also a matter of attitude. A good mental attitude is vital. We can have the best adventure right in front of us, but because of our attitude, it isn't what it could have been. I look at life in a very positive light. I don't think about being positive. For me, it's just a natural state. It's part of the Holy Spirit in me that comes through creating the peace I feel while I'm out on the trail.

When I'm out on the trail, simply getting up in the morning is motivating. I wake up in my tent. The sun maybe coming up. The sounds of the world waking up are all around me. I can't just lay there, not that I want to. I want to get up and I want to get moving. I'm ready to go and I'm excited to see what's in store for the day. That's what motivates me. Being close to the end of a trail can also be a motivator for me. When I get to a certain point in a trail, knowing that I'm within two or three days of finishing; that's motivating.

As for inspiration, I'm not sure what inspires me... God's creation. Man, that's my inspiration! There are times when I have tears in my eyes because of the beauty of what I am looking at. I am in awe about the fact that I have a healthy body. Every day I thank God for the fact that I'm healthy. I'm capable. And He's allowed me to do this.

I'm a person of gratitude. I am so very thankful for life. My signature line reads, "Loving life," after I sign my name. I've done that for years because I do love life. Life is just so full of adventure. Here's my motto: life is an adventure, life is a journey, and life is passion. Adventure, journey, and passion – to me that's life!

The word 'passion' is important. I discuss passion in my talks and stress the importance of discovering your passion. Finding that thing you are passionate about. Maybe you're passionate about hiking and backpacking, raising a family, starting a business, skydiving, whatever it might be... it's important to find your passion. Here are some things to consider: What are you excited about? What steps are you taking to pursue your passion? Are you allowing fear to overshadow, step in, and become a hindrance? I want people to really reflect on those questions.

For me, fear can be another motivator. I think our society is full of fear. We all have our fears, that's a natural part of being human. However, fear, when misplaced, can be a paralyzing emotion which limits our lives. I challenge myself every day to face my fears. When I overcome a personal fear, I learn that it wasn't so bad, and I'm ready to do it again. Overcoming my fears motivates me.

Ultimately though, I am motivated by God's creation. I yearn to be out in the mountains and facing the challenges that lie ahead of me. I love figuring things out...

I have a hard time realizing that I do inspire people. When I think about inspiration, I think about how other people inspire me. It dawned on me recently that I could be that person in the eyes of another person too. So, I can see it from another's perspective.

As you reflect on your accomplishments, what are one or two things that stand out the most for you?

In my mind, I'm just a normal, average, everyday woman. To other people, it may seem that I'm out there conquering the world. But in reality; I'm not. I'm just doing what I love to do and what feels natural to me.

When I first started backpacking, I didn't think about it at all. As the years went by and I began hiking more and more, I started to realize, "Wow, I'm really out here." Of course, that's the big thing – *a female solo hiker.* The number one question I get is, "Aren't you scared?"

When I look back, in my head, I do think, "Wow, I hiked all those miles by myself." Sometimes I'll have a companion on the trail, but for the most part, I am out there solo, a woman hiking by herself. At times, I'll catch myself thinking, "Wow, I forded that river" or "I stayed out by myself" or "I survived that tornado that came through the area" or "I climbed that mountain in the sleet and hail." Taking a moment to reflect on some of the things I have done helps me realize, "Wow, that was me. I did that!"

Last year I completed the New Hampshire 48 Challenge. The Appalachian Mountain Club has designated 48 4,000-foot or higher mountains in New England as a 'peakbaggers' challenge. The task is to 'bag' – hike – all 48 peaks. For me, at my age, that was a huge accomplishment.

Once in a blue moon, I do find myself thinking, "Wow, I've actually hiked from Key West to Maine." I don't track my distance. However, people have told me that over the last few years I have hiked over ten thousand miles. Also, as I get older, I do reflect on all the neat trail experiences I have had. A feeling of accomplishment comes along with the reality that I am a female hiker out there, mostly by myself, enjoying the trails. It's this felt sense of, "Yeah, I've done that!"

If you were to coach a friend, in a similar age range, who was thinking about trying a new sport or wanted to get out there to start moving, what would you tell them?

Unfortunately, a lot of people don't like to exercise; they have little desire to get outside and move. When I talk about getting outside, I can hear the drudgery in people's tone of voice, "Oh, I guess... If you want to go hiking, I can do that" – you can tell it isn't any fun for them.

If someone is completely new to back-packing/hiking, local courses or meet-up groups are a great way to build skills and confidence. I would also suggest joining a local hiking club or find a couple of friends to get out with. If none of the above options were available, I would offer to take them out myself. I would talk to them about how they could begin and help them take some small baby steps toward their goals.

Backpacking/hiking courses are another great way to build skills and confidence. I enjoy working with women and offer courses exclusively for women of all skill and interest levels. Eventually, I'd like to minister to women who have been physically, and/or sexually mistreated/abused. Women who get lost in the shuffle of life. When women are treated unkindly, it has a real impact. Nature is incredibly healing. I know nature has been a huge part of my healing process.

If a woman wants to get outside, but is hesitant, I would encourage her to seek out other like-minded women. During the courses I lead, I often hear women in the group say, "I wouldn't have done this if guys were here." I get the sense that women sometimes feel intimidated or somehow 'weaker' or less capable than the men when it comes to the outdoors. I have noticed that women starting out into the hiking/backpacking world often struggle with a lack of confidence. I have heard women express that they feel "really dumb" at this or that. Sadly, I hear this sort of thing a lot.

On the upside, when women get together in a group, I notice them relaxing. I think it's because they can see other women struggling with the same thoughts and fears. Women are supportive of each other. They can connect with and share the sense of excitement and accomplishment when someone in the group overcomes a fear or learns a new skill.

I know it can be difficult to find other like-minded women. Again, meet-up groups are a good starting point, as are hiking clubs. Nowadays there are lots of companies out there promoting or leading hikes and backpacking trips specifically for women. I would encourage something like that as a first step.

As for first steps to exercising in general... you've just got to get out and do it. GET OUT AND DO IT! That's my motto. I can't stress this enough. Life is an adventure. We're only here for a short period of time. To sit back and watch life pass before your eyes; that's something I am not willing to do. I see life as a journey. We're all writing our own stories. Every day we get to add more detail to the page. When life is all said and done, how do you want that story to look? If you have any desire, please get out and do it. Do not wait until it's too late!

If you had the one piece of sage advice to share with the world what would it be?

To remember that life is precious and that we are blessed with so much. To have a good attitude about yourself, about others, and about life. To remember that we only have this moment. We can't live in the past and we don't know what the future holds. We can't order a redo. Don't walk with regrets. Remember, the only reality is in this moment.

I would also want to say something about Jesus Christ. He's my all in all. Without Him, I wouldn't be here. As I mentioned before, I believe He's given me this platform to be able to speak and to breathe in life and all its wonder. I know when we were together, up on Hanson's Point, I talked about breathing life and encouragement to one another. To remember that our words have power. My prayer for the world would be, "get out there and explore nature; see what a relationship with Him all is about."

Any final thoughts or reflections?

I love the words to this song by the Gaither Vocal Band they sum it up, "Yesterday is gone and tomorrow may never come, but we have this moment today." There is so much truth in that... Yesterday *is* gone, tomorrow *may* never come, but we *do* have this moment today. I say, "Live today with the best possible attitude, with gratitude, and with passion..."

———

ANNIE CRISPINO-TAYLOR

Annie ran her first 100-mile race at 50 years old. Now 60,
Annie has beat cancer and run another ten 100-mile races.

*"You are never too old! If you are patient
enough, you can do it..."*
                                    – Annie Crispino-Taylor

ANNIE, LIKE BUTCH, FOUND ME. Annie responded to a
post I had made in a Facebook group asking to connect
with runners who may be interested in participating in
a 'project'. I knew nothing about Annie; again, I was
happy to let the universe be my guide.

Annie could not be more perfect for this project –
her story has a bit of everything. Annie started
running later in life to relieve some of the stress
related to balancing the responsibilities of family
and child-rearing, with her quest for personal
growth. A dance, I know, many women can relate to.

Annie grew up in California. Not particularly a
'sporty' child in the traditional sense. Horses were
her passion throughout high school. With the
transition to college and adulting, Annie left horses
behind. During college Annie took the opportunity to
travel in Europe for a year, returning to the States in
her early 20s. She took classes here and there, had a

decent job, and worked. Annie married in her 30s. After having three children Annie transitioned into a full-time caregiver role for her three children. When her youngest child was eight, Annie went back to school for her bachelor's degree.

In college Annie found that running, "helped to take my mind off all the studies. I'd take a break and go run." Annie lived near the mountains. Naturally, trail running became a big part of her life. Annie spent countless hours in the mountains with her dog. Annie found running so freeing, "I would go out there, and not think about anything."

At 50 years old Annie ran her first 100-mile race. She then committed to running one 100-mile race every year for the next ten years. In the midst of this Annie was diagnosed with squamous cell carcinoma – an aggressive cancer of the mouth, which resulted in the re-sectioning of her neck and the removal of all her lymph nodes. None of that slowed this woman down. In 2015, fueled by a diet of baby food, Annie ran her scheduled 100-mile race. Annie ran three 100-mile races in 2016. And three more 100-milers in 2017.

As Annie shared her story, I felt humbled, inspired, honored, and incredibly grateful to be able to share Annie's journey. I hope the strength, courage, and tenacity of this remarkable woman shines through her words. Annie's story captures everything this project is about... enjoy!

Annie C

What is your favorite quote or saying?

"Run your own race." I don't know who said it, but I remind myself of this all the time. When I'm running a race or getting caught up in the people around me, this phrase helps me to back off, to focus on me and what I am doing. Using this quote has helped me have a lot more successful races, because I don't get caught up in what other people are doing.

Can you think of a book that stands out in your mind as an influential 'must read'?

I have always loved *To Kill a Mockingbird*. I'm not sure why. There are certain things about the story that really resonate with me. Maybe it's the racial inequities? I lived in the South for a while. Now I live in Portland where there is a focus on racial equality. This topic is close to my heart.

Please share a bit about your background. How did you get interested in this sport, and what were some of your first steps?

My husband and I lived in downtown Sacramento years ago. I was in the area and met some women who happened to be runners. They would often invite me along for a run. Not being a runner, I thought, "Yeah, I'll give it try." So, I tried running a couple of times. Maybe I had the wrong shoes? I'm not sure, but, boy, running hurt my knees like crazy. I decided I didn't like running very much, so I took up cycling instead.

Cycling became my sport. My husband is a cyclist; cycling made sense. I rode bikes for several years, even while raising children. You would often find me with two kids in the bike trailer, and one in the bike seat, heading out for a bike ride. Back then, it was nothing for me to ride 100 miles. That was our routine. When the children got too big for the bike trailer, we progressed to family bike rides. In the summer, we'd go camping and take our bikes along.

When we moved to southern Oregon, my husband joined a local running group. I would tag along and run with the group a couple of times a month. That's when running began to pick up for me. I found a couple of friends who would run with me now and again. I started running during the day. Everyone was working, so I would just head out by myself. I remember, at some point, a girlfriend suggested we run a race together. I said, "OK, let's do it."

I was having so much fun on the trails. As a family we became actively involved in the trail community. I'd head out on the Pacific Crest Trail for a run and also help maintain the trails. At that point, I was doing fun-runs here and there. I can remember a friend encouraging me to do a 50K. I was like, "Nah, nah. I'm good." Back then, I never imagined I would be running 100-mile races.

Tell me about some of the joys, challenges, and milestones along the way.

Currently, I have a friend who's training for a 100-mile race. It's not her first. She's getting back into running after a few years off. I feel a deep sense of satisfaction when she's running her training plan by me. I also feel joy when other runners contact me and ask me for my opinion, when people ask me questions like, "What do you think I should do with my training at this point?" I don't see it as advice, it's more like, "Do you think this is a good idea?" type of discussion. I feel honored when people trust me enough to ask for my input.

Finishing that tenth 100-miler before my 60th birthday – that was a huge joy.

As for challenges, the cancer for sure. Overcoming cancer has been one of the hardest things I have done. Although I did not receive chemotherapy, as my cancer had not spread to my lymph nodes, the daily radiation for six weeks took its toll. After the third week I had developed severe mouth sores and eating became my "job" as my nutritionist put it. But thankfully my husband was by my side, supporting me, making and blending homemade soups with a bone broth base. Although I lost a lot of weight during treatment, I managed to eat enough that I was never required to be tube fed.

Another thing I find difficult is being away from family for long periods of time. My husband used to be a runner. He ran long distances before I ever did. He's very supportive.

Now he is part of the Mount Hood ski patrol team. Coordinating our schedules can be a challenge at times. I do my best to coordinate my long run days with his ski patrol days. That way we can at least have one day over the weekend together. Like all relationships, we both make compromises to support each other with our goals.

Getting to that tenth 100-miler has had its own set of challenges. I completed three before suffering some minor injuries that caused me to DNF three more, then one was canceled mid-race due to bad weather. Then, in 2014, came the cancer diagnosis and treatment. It was after that I decided to resume my goal to get in 10 100-milers before my 60th birthday. I finished the fourth in 2015, and in 2016 completed numbers five and six. However, during my seventh 100-miler attempt I was hit with severe fatigue, which was so bizarre. I made it to mile 68. I just could not continue. After the race, I had some blood work done. They found that I was deficient in iron and vitamin D. Also, my white blood cell count was very low. After some additional testing, I was diagnosed with mononucleosis (mono). Clearly, trying to complete a 100-mile race with mono is not a recipe for success.

Happily, I got through the mono, and some other annoying injuries. I had races seven, eight and nine completed, no problem.

I was ready, prepared, and registered for race number 10 – my final 100-miler before I turned 60. A couple of days before the race, I remember hearing on the news that there were wildfires in the area. Citing safety concerns, the race was canceled. "Ahh, time's running out!" I screamed to myself. With my 60th around the corner, I frantically searched for another race. Thankfully, I found a race in Idaho. I emailed the race director and told them my story. They said, "Yeah sure. Come out and run it." I completed the Idaho 100-miler (IMTUF), my tenth 100-miler, 10 days before my 60th birthday!

Thinking about food as fuel, what have you tried diet-wise? What has been helpful? Are there any supplements you swear by? Do you have any must-have foods when training or competing? What is a treat in your world?

Every day my husband makes me a protein smoothie – mostly fruit, yogurt, and protein powder. Honestly, if he didn't prepare that for me, I know I wouldn't get enough fruit. Because of the cancer, fruit is one of the foods that is very hard for me to eat. Radiation on your head, neck, and especially the mouth area can inhibit saliva production. Thankfully, I have not lost saliva production. In fact, I have the opposite problem: too much saliva. There is something about fruit that just makes my saliva glands go nuts. When blueberries, strawberries, pineapple, and bananas are blended, I can just suck it all down and get three or four servings of fruit in one shot. Whole fruit is difficult for me to swallow.

Another dietary change I have made is the switch to whole milk products. Apparently, whole milk products are better for you because whole milk contains good fat, and the vitamins in milk are fat-soluble. According to the doctors, the vitamins in whole milk products are better assimilated by the body compared with non-fat dairy products. Now I drink whole milk and eat whole-fat yogurt. Although I don't eat that much of it, I do feel like I'm getting more bang for my buck because my body is absorbing all those vitamins.

My breakfast usually consists of a smoothie with some oatmeal and a banana – I eat a lot of bananas. For lunch, I might make some homemade soup. This is another way I get more vegetables into my body. I don't have to blend vegetables, and soup is easy for me to eat. For dinner, we might make chicken and rice with vegetables.

Because of the cancer, I have to eat more frequently. I also have to drink a lot of water with food. The water helps the food go down, but also makes me feel full very fast. I have learned to space my meals out. In a typical day, I eat every two to three hours. Although I get fewer calories per meal, by the end of the day I do get what my body needs.

As for supplements, I take what my doctor prescribes: vitamin D, iron, medication for my thyroid (after radiation my thyroid no longer functions). Other than that, I am not a big fan of supplements. I believe if you focus on a healthy balanced diet, you don't need supplements. As for treats, chocolate! There's nothing better than a chocolate milkshake after a long run.

How did you begin to build your fitness? What were some of your early steps? And how did you know you were starting to form a habit?

For me, my running habit coincided with having a dog. I have a big dog. He has a ton of energy and needs to go out a lot. I enjoy taking him out. Over time, running with the dog became second nature. We have a deal: I make sure I get him out, and he makes sure he gets me out.

When I am training, I usually run at least three days per week with two longer runs on the weekend. During peak training, I run a solid five days, sometimes six days per week. I generally take Monday off and do yoga instead. We have a yoga instructor who comes to our office at lunchtime, which makes it super convenient.

I'm not a morning person, so I tend to run after work. Sometimes I run home from work. It's about a four-and-a-half-mile run, so it's just perfect. Honestly, with the commute, I get home faster when

I run home compared with taking the bus. Once I'm home, I'll grab the dog and we'll run a few more miles. On the weekends, I'll get up early and do my longer runs.

Over the winter, when things slow down, I still run. I may not run as far or as often. I probably have an every-other-day schedule: Tuesday, Thursday, Saturday, and maybe a Sunday run.

Do you have any morning or evening routines?

My routine is pretty strict. I am strict about taking my meds and my eating habits. I take medication every morning, and I eat something every two hours. This starts at 9 a.m. with a smoothie. I eat again at 11 and again at 2 p.m. This routine helps sustain my energy, so I can go for a run in the evening without feeling famished. In the evening, we generally sit down for dinner at around 7 p.m. This schedule seems to work well for me.

Discrimination and/or negativity as an older athlete – do you think this is a thing? Have you personally experienced it? How did you deal with it? What would you tell others?

You know, I hadn't really thought about it. I'm trying to think if there's been a situation where I have felt that sense of, "Oh yeah. That's good for your age" or even that type of attitude. I honestly don't think I have had that experience. Maybe it's because enough people know me and know what I've been through that I don't get treated that way.

Actually, my experience has been the complete opposite. I feel respected. I'm trying to think if I've witnessed this with other women runners. Maybe it's because I haven't talked to people about it. The people I know seem to be inspired by older runners who continue to run well into their 50s, 60s, and 70s. In fact, I get an overall sense of admiration and respect rather than discrimination for older athletes who are still competing and placing in their age categories.

We all have thoughts that can be negative: fears, doubts, that critical voice that might say, "Who do you think you are?" or "What are you thinking? You can't do that." What are some tips and tricks you use to combat your own 'stinking thinking'?

I must admit, it goes back to having that darn dog. That dog that sits there by the front door saying, "I need to get out." Yes, there are days when the last thing I feel like doing is running, but I know that once I put those shoes on and get out the door, I'm going to feel a lot better. Over time, I have learned to recognize that mental state and those limiting thoughts; I know that they will pass.

I have those days when I'm like, "Mm-mm, I'm not gonna run today." A great example: I was putting on my shoes and it was starting to get dark outside and those negative thoughts started creeping in. I remember saying to my husband, "Ah, I think I'll just run tomorrow." I was about to take my shoes off and call it a night when I remembered that my son was coming in for a visit the following day. I knew I wouldn't have the opportunity to run because we would be meeting him for dinner. I remember my thoughts quickly switching to, "Uh oh, I better run tonight, because I won't have a chance to run tomorrow."

My thoughts, which influence my motivation, changed pretty quickly. I put those shoes on, got outside, and did my four and a half miles. I also know that once I get those shoes on and I've been out there for five or ten minutes, all that negativity will go away, and I'll feel so much better.

As for failure, early on in my running career I definitely remember feeling failure. Over time, I have learned how to change my mindset. I ran a race earlier this year. It was a 100-mile race and I didn't finish it. I got to mile 70 and remember the self-doubt was too strong. The race was on the East Coast. It had started to rain – hard. Most of the course, up to this point, had been on the road. I knew the section coming up was going to be the tail and the most technical part of the course. At that point, I was the dead-last runner. There were no sweepers behind me. I didn't know the trail. It was dark, cold, and wet. I decided to stop. Initially, I felt like a failure. I beat myself up with thoughts like, "What's wrong with you? You should have continued."

Deep down in my gut I also had another sense. I felt very uncomfortable and nervous about the circumstances heading into unknown territory, cold, dark, wet, and alone. I made my way to the next aid station where I waited for a ride to the start/finish line. While I was waiting, people were talking about the amount of water on the course. I guess the creeks were overflowing and people were really struggling. I know crossing high water at night is difficult. I didn't have trekking poles to help me make my way across. It would have been impossible to gauge the depth of the water. I recall thinking to myself, "Hmm, good choice." Could I have made it to the next aid station, within the allotted time? Yeah, probably. That's when I start beating myself up again. At some point, I also remember yelling at myself, "OK, look. You made a choice; you just have to be OK with it." Pretty soon, that sense of failure was replaced with feelings of validation and relief: I made the right call.

Most of the time I do OK with failure. Over the years, I have learned to turn it around. I don't say it's failure. I frame it as changing my rules. For instance, if I am working to break a personal record (PR) and it begins to look like that's not going to happen, I change the story. "OK, so today I'm not going to PR. I'm just going to slow down and finish with a good, strong run." I don't consider a change of plan a failure. I realize there are a lot of what-ifs and competitive thinking out there. This comes back to feeling comfortable enough to run your own race. I run races based on my body and my abilities. Over the years, I have learned to be at peace with the decisions I make for myself.

Injuries & illness – have you had any major setbacks health-wise? How do you cope with injuries? Do you do anything to avoid injuries? What tips do you have for healing and recovery?

My only serious illness has been the cancer. I was diagnosed with squamous cell carcinoma on my tongue in January of 2014. In February, I had reconstructive surgery to remove the tumor. They also removed and tested the lymph nodes in my neck, which were all negative for cancer. In March I began six weeks of radiation treatment. The treatments were draining and even after they were complete, my energy was very low. But, speech therapy was an important part of my recovery providing me with tricks for eating and allowing me to gain much of the weight I'd lost within about six weeks. I also had physical therapy to help improve the mobility of my arms, head and neck – the resection surgery to remove the lymph nodes has left me with some mobility limitations, which I continue to treat with daily exercises. The oral surgery has caused slurred speech and some eating limitations, but I have learned to work through those as well.

Last year I was honored to join a special team at the Hood to Coast relay called 'The Cancer Crushers'. A group of mostly women who were either cancer survivors, cancer care givers or both. We were interviewed on the morning news channels, and our photo has been used by Providence hospital in their Finish Cancer campaign. Although I am now five years out from treatment, cancer will always be part of who I am; my 'new' normal.

Thankfully, I haven't been plagued with any major injuries. I'm a believer in catching injuries early. I am also good about getting professional help. I've pulled my hamstring a couple of times. One time, I'm not sure how I did it. I just went out for a run, and two days later I could barely walk. I had the most incredible pain where the hamstring attaches to the butt bone. Off I went to physical therapy (PT). The first round of physical therapy actually made it worse. I don't think they were correctly targeting the point of the injury. Anyway, I wasn't happy, so I found another physical therapist. Thankfully, the second PT had it under control in about a month.

I remember another time I was running when I came across a woman with a puppy. I stopped and we chatted for a bit. Somehow, I got tangled up with her dog. As I moved away, my calf hit the dog in the stomach area. I immediately felt my hamstring tear.

I thought, "Oh man …" I made it back home and put on a pair of super tight compression shorts. I iced and rested the area for about three days. By the time I could get an appointment with the physical therapist, the injury had vastly improved. Needless to say, I am a big fan of compression and ice right away.

I've had some iliotibial band issues in my leg – nothing major – nothing that massage therapy and some strengthening exercises hasn't been able to take care of. I've also had a bout of the dreaded plantar fasciitis (PF). My normal ice-compression routine was not working. The PF plagued me for about six months. I found a chiropractor who specializes in athletes, particularly runners. He's well known for helping many Nike and Olympic athletes get back on their feet. After about four or five visits with him, it was gone. Literally, one day the PF was just gone. I don't know if it was the combination of everything: the months of having various treatments, the strengthening exercises, and the specialized work the PT was doing to loosen up the heel area. Regardless, one day it was just gone. I was like, "Well, I'll take that."

Thankfully, none of the above has been so debilitating that I haven't been able to run. I'm a believer in treating issues as they arise with tools I have learned along the way. So really, that's been it. Of course, as a trail runner, I've had my share of falls, bruises, and scrapes. I broke my finger once after a fall. Overall, I've been lucky. Maybe it's because I'm slow so when I fall I fall in slow motion and the impact isn't so bad.

I'd love to hear about what inspires you... Who are your role models? How do you stay motivated?

I am inspired by other women, particularly runners who are my age or older, people who are still doing some phenomenal things. I realize they may be out of my league, when it comes to some of the things they are accomplishing. Regardless, they still inspire me. I also am inspired by those who work through their struggles, be it poor habits they are trying to break or an illness or injury. I'll think to myself, "If they can do it..." So yes, I may not be able to do the exact same thing, but I can do something similar. Maybe I can't run four 100-milers in 12 weeks, but I could do three 100-milers in a year.

When I am inspired by another person, it generates motivation within me. I start considering the possibilities based on my abilities.

For me, motivation is also linked with habit and joy. I get so much joy out of running. I live near a beautiful park which has access to eight miles of trail. I can lace up, head out the door, run half a mile down the street and I'm in the park. From there, I can see views of Mount Hood. There are great views of the city. You can see all the bridges that span the river. Day or night, it's so beautiful. Having a beautiful place to run inspires me.

I also feel a strong emotional connection to this park. I serve as the race director for an organization, Friends of Mt. Tabor Park. Over the past seven years, our race has raised over $10,000 for the park. Last year, we had two middle school cross-county teams and a Girl Scout troupe participate. This year, over 30 of the 100 participants in the 5K race were under 12 years old. That's incredibly inspiring, and a lot of fun.

As you reflect on your accomplishments, what are one or two things that stand out the most for you?

That's a great question. My first 50K, my first race back after cancer, and my tenth 100-miler for sure. My first 50K was back in 2004. That race was the Siskiyou Outback. This race has always had a special place in my heart. My husband ran his first ultra there. I ran my first ultra there. And, we've volunteered for the race.

The cancer diagnosis came in 2014, almost 10 years to the day after I ran my first 50K. Although I had received the diagnosis, I actually felt fine. I was scheduled to start treatment; like I said, I felt fine, so I signed up for a 50-miler. I thought, "Oh, why not? I'll give it a try."

About halfway through the treatment, I thought, "Oh man. What was I thinking?" I realized I had bitten off more than I could chew. As soon as the treatment was over, I contacted the race directors and explained the situation and that I didn't think I could run the 50-mile distance. The organizers were so gracious... they offered me a choice of three distances: a 15K, a 50K, and the 50 miles. They basically gave me the green light, welcoming me, to come and run any distance I wanted.

About two weeks before the race, I had gone out for a training run with a friend. I remember mapping out the route, thinking it was about 26 miles. We ended up running a whole lot further than we had anticipated. We ran over 30 miles in the scorching heat. It took over nine hours. After we finished, I thought, "If I can do that, then I can run that darn race."

I decided to stay registered for the 50 miles. I headed off to Ashland, Oregon. The race covers part of the Pacific Crest Trail (PCT). The second half of the course involves a lot of climbing. Also, at that time of year, the PCT is busy with thru-hikers making their way from Mexico to Canada. Needless to say, it was a challenging race.

It was my first race back after cancer. I had no idea what to expect. I remember part of a forest section where I was really struggling to make it up a hill. I hadn't eaten enough. I had a Cliff Bar but couldn't get it down – it was too dry. At that point in my recovery, I hadn't worked out the food thing yet.

A couple of PCT hikers cruised past me on that hill. The third person stopped and asked if I was going to be OK. I said, "Yes, I'm fine. I just need to sit here and rest for a minute." I knew the next aid station was about a mile and a half away. I sat for a few minutes, then got back up and made my way to the aid station.

As I reached the aid station, I saw the three hikers happily munching on sandwiches and chips. The volunteers noticed the condition I was in. They threw water over my head and gave me a bunch of fruit to eat. From there, I knew it was only six miles to the finish line. I also knew I'd be fine once I got moving again. Refreshed, I left the aid station. This time, I passed the hikers, joking with them. I said, "Now don't you pass me again."

Of course, my hiker friends did pass me again. Pretty soon the trail started descending, softening into rolling hills. At that point, I was able to run again. I passed the hikers one last time before I headed to the finish line. As you can imagine, that finish was very, very emotional.

If you were to coach a friend, in a similar age range, who was thinking about trying a new sport or wanted to get out there to start moving, what would you tell them?

I would suggest a couple of things. First, keep an open mind and remember making changes in your life is not easy. Then, take baby steps. Find your feet. Experience how your body feels when it's running. Allow your body and mind to adjust. Third, learn to enjoy it before you start competing.

If people are interested in ultra-running specifically, increase your distance slowly. That's how I started. I did a half marathon, then moved up to the 50K distance. I did a 50K one year. Then another the following year. I increased my distance slowly. One year, I felt I was ready for a 50-miler. The year after that, I ran a couple of 50-mile races. By that point, I felt ready for a 100K distance. So, I ran a couple of those. That went well. Then the next logical step was the 100-mile distance. Remember, there's no need to jump into a lot of distance quickly; it's more about the experience.

I know you asked about books… There is a book I read recently called *Run Gently Out There.* It was written by a runner, John Morelock, who has since died. He placed a lot of importance on the concept of learning to run before you start racing.

I hear about so many people picking up this book or trying that training plan and thinking they'll instantly know how to run. Unfortunately, they often end up feeling frustrated or become injured. I believe you must experience running before you can really understand how to run.

Ultimately, that would be my advice to someone starting out. Take it slow. Take the time to really experience running. Learn about your body, how it works, and how it feels. Above all, learn to enjoy running before you even think about competing.

If you had the one piece of sage advice to share with the world what would it be?

That's simple. You are never too old! I truly mean that. I didn't start running until I was pushing 50. If you go about it the right way, if you're patient enough, you can do it, too. Running later in life requires patience, the ability to be OK with who you are, and where you are fitness-wise. Don't compare yourself with others. Learn to be OK with what you can do.

I see a lot of people post, "Oh my run today was horrible." I'm thinking, "Well, what was so horrible about it? What are you comparing it to?" I very seldom come home from a run thinking, "My run was horrible." I accept that every day is going to be different. But I'm very grateful and happy to be able to put my shoes on, to get out there and run.

Finally, be ready to change your perspective midway. If you're going out there with a specific goal, for example, "I'm going to do this in X amount of time," and then halfway through, you're like, "Nah. I'm not feeling it. I'm going to cut back. I'll finish it when I finish it," feel good about it when you're done. Remember, completing a race *is* an accomplishment – even if you are dead last.

Any final thoughts or reflections?

Accept that every day will be different. Celebrate your ability to put on those shoes and get outside to run.

———

PAT GALLANT-CHARETTE

The oldest women to swim the English Channel.

"Sometimes in life the journey is more important than the destination."
— Pat Gallant-Charette

I WAS WORKING ON THE EDITS from Pat's interview during February. As humans we all have what I call seasonal energy shifts. Times when our energy dips and soars. For me, as a writer and an athlete, mid-January to late February is typically a time of year when the parts of my brain that drive motivation and determination struggle to get moving. This year was no exception. I share this because working on Pat's interview gave me the kick in the pants I needed.

Pat was a blast to speak with. Her powerful voice delivered in a rich New England accent leapt off the page. The one thing that came across loud and clear – determination. Pat is one of the most determined people I have ever met. At 67, Pat is an absolute powerhouse when it comes to pushing through 'stinking thinking' and creating a positive mindset. Pat, you are amazing... thank-you!

Pat G

What is your favorite quote or saying?

My favorite quote is from comedian Jonathan Winters. "If your boat doesn't come in, swim out to it." This quote reminds me that you can't let opportunities pass you by. If you see an opportunity, go for it. Although Jonathan passed away some time ago, his words stick with me.

Can you think of a book that stands out in your mind as an influential 'must read'?

I love to read medical journals. I'm a nurse. I have my bachelor's degree in nursing. I enjoy reading about medical things.

Please share a bit about your background. How did you get interested in this sport, and what were some of your first steps?

I came from a big family. I grew up with six brothers and a sister. We all knew how to swim. I was a strong swimmer. During high school, I joined the girls' swim team. Of course, this was back in the early 1960s when they didn't have swim clubs like they have today. Our training was very basic. It literally amounted to a 45-minute swim once or twice a week. We didn't learn how to do flip turns; none of the things a kid would learn today.

After graduating from high school, I went onto

nursing school and qualified as a Licensed Practical Nurse (LPN). I married at 21 and started having children. I went back to school in my early 40s. I graduated from the University of Maine with a bachelor's degree in nursing. By the time I was 46, I was busy working full-time, raising children, and juggling the tasks of family life: groceries, shopping, running kids to sporting events, and all that. I was a typical spectator mom; swimming was the farthest thing from my mind.

Tragedy struck my family. My youngest brother died suddenly of a heart attack. He was 34 years old. Robbie left behind a young wife, a three-year-old son, and a large family who absolutely adored him.

At the time, my 16-year-old son was on the Westbrook High School swim team. Devastated by the loss, my son wanted to swim as a tribute to honor his Uncle Robbie. My brother was a swimmer. Robbie had won the Peaks to Portland, which is a 2.4-mile ocean swim in Maine. I was so touched by my son's desire to honor his uncle, I remember saying, "That's so sweet. I wish I could do the same." My son looked back at me and said, "Well, Ma, you can, if you try."

His response made me take a step back. I saw myself as a spectator mom, not a swimmer. Plus, I hated the ocean and I had a fear of the unknown. Regardless, I decided to give it a try. I promised myself this would be a one-time event.

It took me over a year of training before I was able to qualify for the Peaks to Portland. I remember the day of the swim. I was on Peaks Island with all the other athletes, who, by the way, all looked younger, slimmer, and fitter. There I was, overweight with gray hair, thinking to myself, "What the heck have I got myself into?" Then, suddenly, I calmed down. I remember telling myself, "No, Pat, you can swim this. Who cares if you come in last?" So, I started swimming. The thought, "This is going to be the last time you'll ever do this," kept running over and over in my head.

I knew all those faster, younger swimmers were probably way ahead of me. Somehow it didn't matter. I remember at about the halfway mark, something came over me. A feeling I can best describe as an incredible sense of peace. I was swimming by Fort Gorges, an old domed fort and very scenic area in the middle of the harbor. I could see the lobster boats chugging past me. I could hear the seagulls. It was simply the most gorgeous day. It was in that moment when I fell in love with the sport of open-water swimming.

When I finished, my brother's son was waiting for me at the finish line. We gave each other a big hug. I enjoyed it so much that I decided to enter the race again the following year. I ended up competing in the Peaks to Portland swim for three more years.

Tell me about some of the joys, challenges, and milestones along the way.

At that point, I was in my late 40s. As I headed into my 50s, my thinking had conditioned me to expect physical decline. For me, it was the reverse. I started to get this sense of endurance. Because of my training as a nurse, I knew people could improve a bit, but so drastically? There I was in my early 50s feeling significantly stronger and fitter. I felt like I could swim twice the distance. That was a surprise.

I challenged myself to swim across the Big Sebago, a four-mile stretch of water. I completed that feeling pretty good. I remember telling my husband, "You know, I can go much further than this." So, I set my sights on swimming the two-way crossing of Big Sebago. I trained for another year and completed that swim in a little over seven hours. I finished that swim and felt great. Again, I remarked, "Jeez, I feel as though I can do a lot more. I wonder what I can do next?" My husband suggested, "Why don't you try doing the Channel?" I said, "Oh, OK. That's a great idea!"

I started to do the research. Everything I did was self-taught. I never had a coach. My sons and the high school lifeguard helped me out. They coached me on my stroke and helped me get stronger.

I remember my first English Channel swim attempt. I left the shore feeling totally confident. I had no doubt I could do this. As I got within 1.7

miles of the finish line, I could see the French coast. I could see cars. I could see houses. I was like, "Oh my word, I'm going to get there."

Suddenly, out of nowhere, the tide changed. I immediately started to feel the current pulling me away from France. There's a rule in endurance swimming: if you're not moving forward, you have to end the swim. I argued, suggesting, "Let's swim backward." We had to stop the swim. My first Channel attempt was officially over. Although I was extremely disappointed, I was not defeated. I quickly rebooked for the following year.

With another year of training under my belt, I arrived in England for my second Channel attempt. The whole time we were there we had incredibly high winds. Once again, I returned to Maine. No swim.

I committed to a third attempt and trained hard for another year. My third English Channel swim attempt was slated for 2011. My goal for this attempt was to break the world record for being the oldest woman to swim from Dover to France. The attempt was successful; I made it to the French coast, however, my time fell short of the world record.

I usually dedicate my swims to my brother Robbie by writing his name on my shoulder. I had another brother, Johnny, who died when he was 17 after a tragic accident in high school. I like to dedicate my English Channel swims to my deceased brothers by writing their names on my shoulders.

At the age of 66, I tried again. This time I set the world record. I became the oldest woman to swim solo across the English Channel. My son Tom was there as part of the crew. It was truly a heartfelt moment having Tom there to witness my world record – an incredible joy!

Thinking about food as fuel, what have you tried diet-wise? What has been helpful? Are there any supplements you swear by? Do you have any must-have foods when training or competing? What is a treat in your world?

Many years ago, when I started this journey, there was not much information about nutrition for marathon swimmers. I remember looking to the ultra-running community for advice. I wanted to know how people were running 50 and 100 miles. What were they doing for hydration? How were they sustaining their energy? What products were they using? I'd just buy the same products and experiment with them. I've probably tried everything on the market.

For a while, I was using a lot of those carb mixes, specialty drinks, and sports gels. I got to the point where, by about 10 hours into a swim, I was literally vomiting after using those products. During my last marathon swim, I told my crew, "Please, no more. Just give me a bottle of water and a peanut butter cookie." That's all I need.

The peanut butter cookie gives my body enough

calories to swim for an hour and the water takes care of the hydration. So, that's my grand nutrition plan. A peanut butter cookie or some crackers and a bottle of water once every hour. Simple and effective. No more getting sick. Plus, I feel great.

Supplements-wise, I take Osteo Bi-Flex. I have had some issues with one of my hips. I tried a stationary bike for the first time and overdid it, causing some discomfort in my hip. A friend told me about Osteo Bi-Flex, so I started using that. I also take calcium with vitamin D. That's about it.

As for favorite foods or treats, I usually don't have any appetite after I finish a swim. Like most marathon swimmers, swimming in saltwater makes my tongue get covered in a white coating and swells. After I swam Molokai's 26-mile channel in Hawaii, my tongue was almost pure white – I couldn't eat anything. The only way I could hydrate was with a straw pointed at the back of my throat. After about 24 hours, my tongue started healing and I was fine. Generally, after a 24-hour swim or a long marathon swim, I have no interest in food. I do drink a lot of fluids to rehydrate.

How did you begin to build your fitness? What were some of your early steps? And how did you know you were starting to form a habit?

I remember when I first started to get back into swimming, it took me a long time before I could swim even 30 minutes without stopping. I had to slowly start to build my stamina. Remember, I didn't have a coach or a trainer, so, again, I looked at the marathon running community. I wanted to know how they trained to run 26 miles.

Let's take an average marathon runner's week. A runner might schedule short runs on Sunday, Monday, Tuesday, Wednesday. On Thursday, they might increase their distance a bit. On Friday, it's a short run again. The weekends would be days when the long runs were scheduled.

I thought, "Wow, if it works for them, it must work for swimmers, too." So, I followed a similar schedule. My training plan consisted of an easy 30-minute swim with a slow build up to an hour swim. On my day off from work, I would do a long swim, maybe an hour and 15 minutes. Every two weeks, I slowly increased my time in the water. I would do an hour swim on Sunday, Monday, and Tuesday with a long two-hour swim on my day off. With this schedule, over time, I was able to increase the length of my swims. Before long, I was able to do some very long swims.

Another training method ultra-marathoners use is back-to-back running: running two longer runs in two days. I took that concept and added back-to-back swims into my training schedule. I did my short swims during the week. On Saturday, I would swim for three hours. Then on Sunday, I would head out and swim for four hours. Apparently, this method tricks your body into thinking you did a full seven-hour swim, even though in reality, you were splitting it up. This is how I trained for the English Channel. Although this was a popular training method in the ultra-running community, I was not convinced this method would work for swimming. However, I was willing to give it a try.

In training for the English Channel, the longest training swim I did was a 10-hour swim off the coast of Maine followed by a five-hour swim the following day. This was my final big swim a month before my first attempt.

The day of my first English Channel swim attempt, I swam for 16 hours and 43 minutes. I had never swum that far in my life. However, my body felt as though I had done it before – it felt accustomed to doing it. I attribute this to the back-to-back swims.

I think it's important to mention that I didn't use the back-to-back method every week. I gradually built up to this over a year. Let's say I started training in January, I would do a back-to-back swim: three hours followed by four hours one weekend in January. The following month, I would increase it by an hour. And then the following month, by another hour. It wasn't like people were saying, "Oh my God, you just did a 10-hour swim!" I did longer back-to-back swims once a month. That seemed to be enough to register in my body that I could do that distance.

Plus, I had full confidence. People often comment, "Wow, I didn't know you could swim that far." Of course, people don't see all the baby steps I have taken along the way.

Naturally, I have made mistakes; that's part of a learning process. One example of a mistake is when I used a stationary bike for the first time. I figured, I'm an endurance athlete. I can do two hours on a stationary bike, easy. Boy, was I wrong! I ended up with tendonitis in my legs.

Later, I was telling someone in the gym what happened, and they said, "Jeez, you're only supposed to do, like 15 to 20 minutes for your first time ever." I was like, "All righty, now, I don't have a coach, you know?" I definitely won't make that mistake again.

Do you have any morning or evening routines?

As routines go, every day is different. I am retired from nursing and I am my grandchildren's full-time babysitter. My daughter is a nurse. She works the 4 p.m. to 4 a.m. shift. When she gets home from work, she needs to sleep. Of course, the kids' schedule is dictated by the school year. They are either at school or on a break. Either way, I take care of the children when she is at work. You know the routine – kids come home from school. I help with homework. We have supper. Then it's bedtime. In the morning we get them up and do it all over again.

Now I'm retired, I can work my training around the kids' schedule. I generally swim five days a week. Some days, it's an hour, sometimes it's an hour and a half, sometimes it's two hours – it varies. When I am training, I swim six days a week.

Two years ago, I made a list of things I wanted to do. One of my bucket list items was to do more arts and crafts with my grandchildren. One Saturday the grandkids came over and we sat and did arts and crafts all day long. After sitting for a while, I got up to walk across the kitchen. I felt like I was a hundred years old. I could barely walk. All my joints had stiffened up from sitting for so long. I quickly realized the importance of movement. Now, if I'm doing arts and crafts with the grandchildren, I'll sit for an hour then I'll get up and move. For me, that's usually a brisk walk outside to get some fresh air – I just can't sit down all day. Needless to say, regular movement throughout the day is a huge part of my routine.

Discrimination and/or negativity as an older athlete – do you think this is a thing? Have you personally experienced it? How did you deal with it? What would you tell others?

Yes, I have experienced it. Years ago, when I realized I had the ability to be a marathon swimmer, I mentioned it to a couple of people. I remember being at a pool talking about my hopes with a group of swimmers, thinking they'd be supportive. I clearly remember one of the people literally laughing in my face. Then there was another incident when an older gentleman laughed at me as he shook his head and said, "You do not know what you're getting yourself into."

I'll tell you; I often think of those two people when I am reaching a finish line or have won a world record. When I encounter negativity, I have to turn it around. I acknowledge that, yes, they have their own opinion, but they don't know me, my drive, or my determination. When I'm in the middle of a tough swim, I think of them. In my head, I'm like, "OK, I can do this. And I'm going to show you I can do this."

But, of course, there's always chatter in people's heads about reaching a certain age and doing, or not doing, a certain thing. I can see how some people might think that way. Years back, when I was in my 40s, I didn't know any 67-year-old marathon swimmers. Most marathon swimmers were retiring in their 40s or 50s, not at 67! Looking back, I admit, I had the same kind of thoughts. But now I am older, I have a bit more wisdom. I believe people should do what they want to do in life and just go for it. Don't be limited by society's constraints and conditioning about age, aging, and being too old to try something new. I tell people, as long as they feel healthy, they feel strong, and they're willing to work, then go for it. Remember, you're never too old.

When I worked full-time as a nurse on my feet all day, there were many times I felt like going home after a long shift, crashing on the couch, and turning on the news or watching Oprah. But I didn't. I went straight from work down to the beach and swam for an hour. The thing is, I felt more relaxed during that swim.

After being on my feet all day, all I wanted to do was lie down. Technically, when I was swimming, I was lying down and my feet were up. I remember feeling such enjoyment being in that water. I felt energized. Leaving work, heading down to the harbor, and going for a swim even if it was just for an hour became an important part of my routine. To me, swimming after a hectic day felt so much better than coming home, turning on that TV, and crashing on the couch.

We all have thoughts that can be negative: fears, doubts, that critical voice that might say, "Who do you think you are?" or "What are you thinking? You can't do that." What are some tips and tricks you use to combat your own 'stinking thinking'?

I am the queen of negative thinking. When I swam the English Channel at the age of 66, I remember my first few steps into the water off the English coast. The water temperature was so cold. Immediately, I found myself saying, "Oh, Pat, this is going to be a long day. You're never going to be able to make it to

France in this water temperature." The water temperature was in the low 50s. Then I said to myself, "OK, Pat, stop with the negative thinking. Wait until the sun comes up. By about 10 a.m., you're going to feel the warmth from that sun. And you'll be glad you stayed in."

Well, 10 o'clock came, the sun came up – I wasn't feeling any warmer. I started with the negative thinking again. It was like, "Oh my God, I can't quit after four hours. Just go two more hours." Then I started telling myself, "OK, Pat, think positive thoughts. You can do this. You can do this. You can do this." Six hours into the swim, I was cold and combating this negative thinking. At about the halfway point, I told myself, "Look, the worst is behind you. Start thinking more positive. The water temperature will get warmer the closer you get to France."

As I got closer to France, the water wasn't any warmer. The negative thinking started up all over again. I remember saying in my head, "Oh my word, when is this swim going to be over?" That started another round of me having a good talking to myself. "Pat, stop with this negative thinking. Think positive. You're three-quarters of the way there. You've got to hang in there. You're almost there. Stop with this negative thinking." This back-and-forth routine continued on and on in my head. Then, all of a sudden, I looked up and there was the beach – France!

I swear, during that swim, 80% of my thoughts were negative. I thought about quitting countless times. The same thing happened with the Molokai swim. In the middle of the night, I got bumped pretty hard – the crew thought maybe a dolphin had struck me in the leg; I felt like quitting right there. The kayaker encouraged me, "You know, Pat, the worst is behind you. Wait until the sun comes up. You'll change your mind." I continued swimming with my mind sputtering with all this negativity. Of course, he was right, as soon as that sun came up, I felt a huge turn in my thoughts and pure determination kicked in.

It's also natural to have self-doubts. I had them on my very first Peaks to Portland swim. I felt intimidated by being surrounded by all these young, slender athletes. I remember having to tell myself, "You know, Pat, just calm down. You can do this. You've trained for it. You have every right to be here." It would be different if, for example, I got to England ready to swim the Channel with absolutely no training. Then yes, I'd have every reason to have negative thoughts and doubts. But when you know you've put the time in, you know you've trained in the right way, when those negative thoughts start trickling in, you've got to put them on the back burner. Recognize what they are: only thoughts. Put them aside and keep moving forward.

Here's a great example from my early years

about how I learned to not listen to my negative thoughts. I was training at Pine Point Beach, a popular coastal beach in Maine. My intention was to do a three-hour swim that day. Well, about an hour and a half in, I started to feel like I was getting too cold. Nothing major, no hypothermia or anything. Anyway, my mind was saying, "You know, Pat, you've had a long week. Nursing has been so hard this week. It's Saturday. Let's just jump out [of the lake] and enjoy the day. Plus, you know you're getting very cold." All these negative thoughts were flooding my mind.

I listened to that stinking thinking, stopped swimming, and got out of the water. I was out of the water for about five seconds. I wasn't the least bit cold. It was my thoughts telling me I had to stop. In reality, I wasn't tired. I wasn't cold. Yet, I stopped and got out of that water. I said to myself, "Pat, you're listening to those negative thoughts. And you fell for it." Right there, I made a deal with myself, unless my body is actually having symptoms of hypothermia, I am not to listen to that negativity. From that experience, I have learned to ignore negative thinking and keep moving forward to the finish line.

I have also learned that there is a difference between listening to your body and listening to your thoughts. I wasn't feeling cold, yet my thoughts were telling me I was dangerously cold. I had none of the physical symptoms. I wasn't shivering. My fingers weren't separating. I wasn't getting any finger cramps. I had absolutely no symptoms. It was my head telling me, quit, quit, quit. Just go home and have a nice relaxing day.

Of course, hypothermia can be very dangerous. Since then, my crew has been trained to recognize symptoms of hypothermia. It still blows me away that negative thoughts can be so powerful that they tricked me into thinking I was experiencing physical symptoms of hypothermia.

Believe me, there are those times when I find myself thinking, "You know, Pat, just take the day off, you've swam four days in a row." Then, I would stay home, and it was like, "Jeez, why didn't I get out there?" I am annoyed with myself because it was a perfectly beautiful day to swim and the following day was raining and cold.

Sometimes I push myself. However, I firmly believe in listening to your body. If you truly feel tired one day, take a day off from the sport that you love. Go for a walk or do something else instead.

Injuries & illness – have you had any major setbacks health-wise? How do you cope with injuries? Do you do anything to avoid injuries? What tips do you have for healing and recovery?

About three years ago, I was swimming in the ocean. There was a bad storm occurring to the south of us. Even though where we were it was a nice sunny day, the swells were getting bigger. I am not a deep-water swimmer. I like to swim in waist or chest level water. Anyway, I was swimming along when out of nowhere this huge wave crashed over me. I plummeted right to the bottom of the ocean and hit my shoulder. I oriented myself, brushing it off thinking, "Oh, it's nothing," and started swimming again. I finished my swim, got out of the water, and went home. The next day my shoulder was very sore.

To make a long story short, I had damaged my shoulder. I ended up having surgery to repair the damage, which put me out of commission for a while. I followed doctor's orders. I went through rehab. Within 10 months, I was healed and back to marathon swimming.

The shoulder surgery taught me to really listen to what the rehab specialist had to say. I knew someone who had a similar surgery. They didn't do the exercises like they were supposed to, and they ended up with a lot of problems.

After my shoulder surgery, I wanted to get back into the pool as quickly as possible. I asked my doctor when I could swim again. He was dismayed, reminding me, "You can't use your arm to swim." I suggested, "How about I keep my arms at my side and just kick?" He gave me the thumbs-up. Yes, I had to wait for the small incisions to heal, but I was back in the pool within a week. I swam on my back with my arms at my side. I used my legs more. I was careful not to use that arm until they gave me the all-clear.

Even though the shoulder was very painful, I pushed myself and followed exactly what the doctor ordered. I had the best recovery. I tell everyone, if you have a surgery or some type of injury, follow to the T your doctor's orders.

I also recognize that burnout can be a problem. I know several swimmers who have struggled with burnout and they have just quit. They train, train, train – not giving themselves enough time to rest. After a big event or a marathon swim, I treat myself. I give myself permission to take the next two to three weeks off. I don't go into the water. I'll plan some fun activities. Maybe go out to lunch with some friends. Go shopping or do other things I enjoy. When it's time to get back in the pool, I feel energized. I love this sport. It's like I haven't missed a beat.

I'd love to hear about what inspires you… Who are your role models? How do you stay motivated?

I would say my son has inspired me the most with the words he said to me all those years ago. There are also other marathon swimmers I greatly admire. For instance, Jackie Cobell from the United Kingdom. Jackie holds the world record for the longest time to swim from England to France. After swimming for 28 hours, she made it! Jackie may not be the fastest swimmer, but she's determined, she puts the time in, and she knew she could do it. People like Jackie inspire me. People who are really dedicated to their sport also inspire me. People who put in the time regardless of age, or speed, or what others think, inspire me. That kind of desire and determination I find incredibly inspirational. Jackie, who is in her 60s, has recently progressed to ice swimming. She goes all over the world competing in ice swimming championships. I admire her determination and her grit.

As you reflect on your accomplishments, what are one or two things that stand out the most for you?

That's a hard question to answer because there's so many of these swims. They're all unique. For me, it's not so much about the accomplishments, it's more about the journey and the learning. Believe me, I've had plenty of failures. I have learned how to accept them and keep moving forward. I've seen people get so frustrated and disheartened by 'failure' that they quit. I have done so many swims that were not successful. I think that's the thing I reflect on the most; it's about determination. In life, sometimes things don't go the way you want them to. You can't give up. You've got to keep pursuing the thing you enjoy. I think my biggest accomplishment has been about building determination.

If you were to coach a friend, in a similar age range, who was thinking about trying a new sport or wanted to get out there to start moving, what would you tell them?

I would tell them to go slow and not to go overboard. I have met people who want to start running. They go out super hard that first week. Then they get shin splints and they're out of commission for the next two months. Just go slow.

It's the same for walking. Yes, you've got to get out and start somewhere. If you've been a couch potato, build up slowly. Start with a five-minute walk in the morning, 10 minutes in the afternoon, and another five minutes in the evening. Break a 20- or 30-minute walk into smaller chunks.

Whether you are running, walking, or cycling, allow your body to adjust. It takes time. Be patient. Then slowly begin to increase your distance. Before you know it, you'll reach the point where you're comfortably exercising once a day or twice a day. Go easy. Don't try to run a marathon your first week out. When I started swimming, I remember feeling so proud and accomplished after I finished my first hour-long swim. I felt like I had won a gold medal! Take time to enjoy the journey.

Believe me, it took me a long time before I was able to swim for one hour nonstop. Now, 21 years later, I can swim 24 hours nonstop, no problem. It's because I slowly built up the endurance. I think that's how a lot of people in our age bracket – 50s,

60s, and 70s – get injured. People want to make positive changes, but they overdo it. Take baby steps. Mix it up. Do something different every day. Go for a walk one day, take the next day off. Try cycling. Then take a day off. Go for a swim. Then take the next day off. Before you know it, you'll build that stamina. Remember to have some fun along the way.

That's how I did it. I have an old-fashioned bike like the ones I grew up with in the '50s. I still can't figure out how to operate all those gears on one of those specialty bikes. I would take the grandkids out, and we'd have a ball. Then the following day, I would go for a half-hour walk. The next day, I'd go for a swim.

Try not to get caught up in the competition, like riding a stationary bike for two hours straight – that was a big mistake! If you take the time to build up slowly, you'll be amazed at what your body can do.

If you had the one piece of sage advice to share with the world what would it be?

To live your life because you never know which way the road is going to go. And be willing to try something new. Find something you like. You might discover a road that you never imagined.

Take my case. I never, ever imagined that I would be a marathon swimmer. Never. I tried something new and was stunned to find that I was able to swim long distances. If someone has an opportunity to try something new – it doesn't have to be a sport – go for it! It could be dancing or something artistic. No matter, you may find that it takes you on a journey that you just never, ever imagined.

Here's a good example of that. I had a swimsuit company from New York contact me and ask if I wanted to be a swimsuit model. They flew me to California. I was in a photo shoot with Brooke Shields and Ashley Graham. And I'm thinking, "Sheesh, I'm 67 years old, overweight, with gray hair. They want me to be a swimsuit model?" Again, you just don't know where life is going to take you. You've got to be open to the adventure.

This journey of mine has been incredible. Swimming has brought so much joy and richness to my life. Swimming has taken me all over the world. I have met so many incredible people. It's honestly been an unbelievable experience.

Any final thoughts or reflections?

Maybe for some of the working parents and grandparents out there: when I started marathon swimming about a decade ago that was also about the same time that I started babysitting my grand-children. I have three grandchildren. The oldest one is 10. Over the past 10 years, I have babysat all three of them. At that time, I was still working full-time as a nurse. I'd get out of work at 3:30 and be at my daughter's house by 4 to watch the kids overnight. I'd get up and go back to work the next day. The days I didn't have to babysit was the time I did my swimming.

My point is, don't let life, time, work, and schedules get in the way of your dreams. Although I was working and babysitting my grandchildren every week, I still found time to train. I capitalized on my days off from work. Those would be my long training days. The days I was babysitting – at one time I had two in diapers and a toddler – I'd bundle them up, put the babies in the carriage and the toddler would walk. I can't tell you how many times we walked back and forth up and down the drive-way. It was like, OK, I can't go swimming, but I still need to exercise for an hour after I got home from work. So, that's what I did.

As the grandkids got older, we would go to the park. They would play. I'd keep my eye on them as I walked around the playground. We would do that for an hour or so. They would get outside, and I would get my exercise for the day.

I want to encourage anyone who feels like they don't have time to exercise, maybe due to work and family responsibilities, please, make the time. To stay active is so important for your health. If you reach your 60s and 70s and you've never done any exercise, your body will get weaker so much faster.

On the other hand, if you stay active, it will keep you stronger mentally and physically when you are well into your 60s and 70s.

Finally, you also have to figure out how to stay active in the off seasons. Here in Maine, it's too cold to swim in the ocean in the winter. Of course, I use an indoor pool. But I miss the fresh, cool outdoor air.

I remember one winter when we built the grandkids an old-fashioned ice-skating rink in the backyard. My husband built up banks of snow so we could sled down onto the ice. Again, this was keeping me busy and active instead of sitting on the couch watching TV. At 4 o'clock when my daughter headed out to work, the kids and I would go out and play in the snow. One year we put up Christmas lights so we could skate in the dark. The kids loved it. We all loved it! Staying active is the key to staying healthy and healthy aging. I certainly don't feel 67.

———

DAN TAYLOR

'Ran two marathons per year between the ages of
70 and 80 years old. At 85 he's still rockin'...'

"Listen to your body and don't overdo it."
– Dan Taylor

SPEAKING WITH DAN was like having a conversation with a living breathing running historian. He has a depth of knowledge that goes back to the early 1970s when the New York Marathon cost a $1 to enter and fewer than 200 people showed up to compete. For comparison, the same race in 2017 had a price tag of $295 and 100,000 lottery applications. Over that half a century Dan has experienced, first-hand, Apartheid in South Africa, kidnapping in South America, conflict in China, and a rattlesnake bite – all through the eyes of a runner.

Dan has run in countries all over the world and competed in countless marathons. In his seventh decade Dan ran two marathons a year. Dan explains that, "It's easier to stay in shape than to get back into shape." Dan, now 85 years old, sees running as a vital part of his mental, physical, and social health.

Dan, like the other amazing athletes in this book, was not 'famous' and didn't know me from a hole in the ground. Dan's name came up in a thread when I was looking for my last two interviewees. Someone mentioned that, "there's a guy out there in his 80s who just ran the Boston Marathon." I thought, "That's a guy I want to talk to." I did a bit of digging and chased him down. I am thankful and honored to be able share Dan's *extra*-ordinary story with you. Enjoy!

Dan T

What is your favorite quote or saying?

I don't have one. Not that I can think of. Now, I might think of it as soon as I hang up. It's amazing how memory comes and goes when you are my age.

Can you think of a book that stands out in your mind as an influential 'must read'?

Jim Fixx's book, *The Complete Book of Running*. Jim was a runner who died running a marathon. Jim wrote a great book about running, which is now part of his legacy. There's also a book called *A Race Like No Other: 26.2 Miles Through the Streets of New York*, written by Liz Robbins, who is a staff member at the *New York Times*. In the book, Liz describes the New York City Marathon and the wonder of running through all five boroughs of New York City. The course winds through the Bronx, which is heavily African American. Then you run through

Hasidic Jewish communities, with their long braids, and black costumes. She describes the incredible range of diversity within the various communities. Of course, New York City and the New York City Marathon are like no other. Liz does a great job with describing the race and all its glory.

Please share a bit about your background. How did you get interested in this sport, and what were some of your first steps?

At 32 years old, I was a pack-a-day smoker. I was 202 pounds. And, I rarely got off the couch. A part of me knew that if I didn't change my ways, I was headed for an early grave. The first thing I did was quit smoking. Quitting smoking was probably the hardest thing I have ever done. It took me 10 years to completely stop. As part of the 'new me' I drastically changed my eating habits and I started running. I didn't run far, just around the block.

As a kid, I was never involved in track or cross-county running. I didn't have any background in running. This was all new to me. I started out with very short walks around the block. Once I was comfortable with walking, I began to run around the block. As my activity and stamina increased, my weight decreased. Pretty soon, I lost 50 pounds and was able to run farther. When I turned 45, 12 years later in 1978, I signed up to run the New York City Marathon for the first time. This was the second year of the race and it was held on a new course. The new course started in Staten Island, winds through all five boroughs of New York City, ending in Central Park. It was absolutely unbelievable.

Way back then, there weren't many people running marathons. You just signed up and they let you in. I completed my first New York Marathon with a time of three hours and 53 minutes, my best time ever for any marathon I have ever run. At 45 years old, I was hooked. Running became my thing.

Honestly, I have lost count of all the marathons I have run over the past 40 years. Naturally there have been periods when I couldn't run marathons. I had pneumonia once and I've had a couple of minor surgeries. Interestingly, to this day, I have never had any joint issues or problems with my knees, ankles, or my hips. People ask me all the time, "Don't you wear anything out?" My standard response: "I don't believe you *wear* out. I believe you *rust* out."

In my mind, rusting out is created by a sedentary lifestyle. When you spend your time sitting on the couch, before you know it, you've gained 50 pounds and you've got a bad knee, a bad hip, or some other ailment. Anyway, I wasn't willing to rust, so I kept running.

Tell me about some of the joys, challenges, and milestones along the way.

It's funny, when I was younger, people would ask me all the time, "Are you going to run the Boston Marathon?" I'd reply, "No. I'm too young." They'd say, "Too young! What do you mean?" "Well," I'd explain, "you have to qualify for Boston; the older you get, the slower you can run to qualify." At this point, I think I've run nine Boston Marathons.

When I reached 70, I told myself that I would have to run two marathons a year to stay in shape. For me, getting back in shape is far more difficult than staying in shape. I am proud to say that between the ages of 70 and 80, I ran 20 marathons, completing my goal of running two marathons a year.

My spring marathon was the Boston Marathon. My fall marathon would be either the Wineglass Marathon located in Corning, New York, the New York Marathon, the Philadelphia Marathon, or the Virginia Beach Marathon. I like the Virginia Beach Marathon; it's held around St. Patrick's Day and run on a flat course using a figure-eight loop. If the wind's coming in one direction, you get the benefit of it half the time and fighting it for the other half of the time.

When I turned 80, I celebrated by running the Boston Marathon. I wasn't at all sure that I would be ready for the 2014 Boston Marathon. In December, the previous year, I had a compression fracture in my twelfth vertebrae and a case of pneumonia. I was actually seeded second in my age division – there aren't that many people running at that age. Nonetheless, I was seeded second and completed in an acceptable time to be on record as an official finisher. I am particularly proud of this accomplishment.

The Boston Marathon is always the third Monday in April – Patriots' Day. I was incredibly determined to compete in the 2014 Boston Marathon because it was the year after the bombing took place. I remember the day of the bombing. I was having a difficult race that year due to some health issues. My wife and daughter always accompany me to the Boston Marathon, typically they see me at the mile 21-22 marker, then they head down, with the crowd, to welcome the finishers across the finish line.

When they tried to do this in 2013, the police wouldn't let them through. The area was cordoned off, police were stopping people and turning them away. At that point, they had no idea what had happened. If I had been running at my usual pace, my wife and daughter would have been standing right across the street from where the bombs exploded. I have never felt so fortunate to have a bad day.

To be an official finisher of the Boston Marathon, you must complete the race in six hours. That year [2013], I finished in five hours and 54 minutes. I made the cutoff by six minutes. So, that's been my running career.

I am currently 85 and still running. I ran an hour today. I'm not as fast as I used to be. I follow the

Galloway system. Jeff Galloway has a system where you intersperse some walking with the running. For instance, in a 26.2-mile race, you would walk a minute for every 10 minutes you run. This way you are not collapsing at the end. For my run today, I ran for two minutes and walked for three. Sometimes, I will run for three minutes and walk for two. It just depends on how I feel.

I used this method to run a virtual Boston Marathon. If for some reason I can't physically make it to the Boston Marathon, I run it virtually. With this method, you run your 26.2 miles wherever you are. You can walk. You can run. You can run-walk. You can do whatever you like. The good news is that you are the only person doing it. There are no qualifying times, no cutoff times. You're competing against yourself. If I get my 26.2 miles completed during daylight hours, then that was my goal. For me that's a win!

As you get older, you experience a lot of changes. My wife of 60 years passed away a couple of years ago. I miss her and get depressed from time to time. I have found that getting up in the morning and going for a run or doing any exercise – maybe the stationary bike or lifting weights – lifts my mood and I feel much better. If all I did was sit around, eat, mope, and feel sorry for myself, I don't know where I would be.

Along with keeping my mental health and my

weight in check, another joy related to running is that all three of my kids run. They don't run marathons. They'll split up a marathon between them, each running part of the way with me. All my children run regularly; now, some of my grandchildren run, too. Running is a huge part of my life. That's all there is to it...

Thinking about food as fuel, what have you tried dietwise? What has been helpful? Are there any supplements you swear by? Do you have any must-have foods when training or competing? What is a treat in your world?

Food-wise, I don't like to have a lot in my system before a race. I might eat a baked potato with a small hamburger the night before. On race day, I swear by Power Bars. I take Power Bars and break them into six small pieces. After the first mile, I'll eat a bit, then a bit more, and then some more. I find that's just enough to keep my energy up. I am also a big Gatorade fan.

As for supplements, I take vitamin D occasionally. I was diagnosed with peripheral neuropathy a while back. Peripheral neuropathy (PN) is a tingling sensation in your extremities. People get it in their hands and toes. For some people, it can be extremely painful. Thankfully, for me, it's not that bad. My doctor prescribed B12 to help with the PN, so I also take a B12 vitamin every day.

I started seeing a cardiologist when I was 70. He examines me every year. He gives me the thumbs-up to run. In the last couple of years, he's not been particularly enthusiastic about my running habits. Per doctor's orders, I take a baby aspirin every day. I also take the smallest dose of a statin that you can possibly take. That's part of my cardiology regime and keeps the doc happy.

After a race, when your whole body is screaming, getting a massage is a real treat. Some of the marathons I've run had massages available for finishers – that's absolutely wonderful! I also like the little bottle of wine they give finishers at the Guthrie Wineglass Marathon, located in the heart of the Finger Lakes in New York. I am never sure whether to drink the wine or not; I don't want to be staggering around. Generally, after a race I am not that hungry. I may have a small post-race snack. After I have recuperated a bit, my family and I head out to celebrate. One of my absolute favorite restaurants is in Boston. This restaurant has the best planked salmon. That's always a treat!

How did you begin to build your fitness? What were some of your early steps? And how did you know you were starting to form a habit?

You know, I'm not sure when that was. Pretty early on, I remember feeling this great sense of accomplishment, that feeling of setting a goal for yourself.

In my head, I was saying, "I'm going to run 10 miles today." You go out and measure the route. Then you run it. No matter where I am in my running journey, for me, that felt like an incredible feeling of accomplishment. I also love the feeling of euphoria when I cross the finish line.

When I first started running, I started out with small steps. I would literally head out with the intention of making it around the block. I would walk a bit and run a bit, walk a bit and run a bit. I did my block routine regularly. Over time, I slowly built my stamina and found that I was also able to increase my distance.

The first steps are always the hardest. Even today, after running for close to 50 years, the hardest step is the first step. Now, for me, it's those first six miles or so. After mile six, it gets easier and easier. You've got to push through those first steps. Trust me, it will get better.

I have heard a lot of people say they get to about the four-mile mark and can't run anymore. If you have a significant ache or pain, or you're injured, then of course you should stop. If your body is fine, then you have to push through – this is a mental barrier. Once you push through that mental barrier, you'll find, over time, that your breathing will start to balance. This restores the oxygen to your muscles. Pretty soon, you notice all the systems in your body – breathing, muscles, brain – getting in sync. When it kicks in, you'll know it. You'll feel like a running machine.

As for my current training schedule, I still follow Jeff Galloway's system. I take one day off a week. The rest of the week, I run and cross-train. For example, I will go up to the exercise facility, ride a stationary bike for 30 minutes or so, then I lift weights. At this point in my life, I'm not interested in building muscle. I just want to keep the muscle I have. I alternate time in the gym with a six- or eight-mile walk-run, as long as the weather is decent.

Do you have any morning or evening routines?

I almost always run and exercise in the morning. I find that if I am up and running it helps with any depression I might be having due to my late wife's demise. I feel much better for the rest of the day.

Discrimination and/or negativity as an older athlete – do you think this is a thing? Have you personally experienced it? How did you deal with it? What would you tell others?

Actually, no. I can't tell you how many people have said what an inspiration I am. When you're 70, 75, 80 years old and you're still running marathons, people are very congratulatory. I get comments like, "Oh, God. I could never do that." You just don't know what you are capable of until you try.

Running culture has changed a lot over the past 50 years. When I first started running years ago, I vividly remember times when I was out running, and the local school bus would pass me. Kids would throw Coke bottles out of the windows at me because they thought I was crazy. You just didn't see people running on the roads. Back then only 'crazy people' ran.

In places you might expect some negativity or judgement; it has turned out to be the complete opposite experience. I remember visiting Malawi in southern Africa when I traveled for work. Back then, it was unusual to see a white face, let alone a white face running. The local people just looked and smiled. They nudged whoever they were with as if to say, "Look at that guy," with nothing but interest and curiosity.

At home, I would run on the local high school track. One winter, I was running on the track when a skiff of snow came through. When I went back to the track the next day, my solo footprints were still there. I was the only one using the track.

Interestingly, a decade later, when I left Charleston, West Virginia you almost had to have a ticket to get on the track. I'm exaggerating a bit, but the point is that the concept of running for pleasure or exercise seemed to explode over that 10-year period.

We all have thoughts that can be negative: fears, doubts, that critical voice that might say, "Who do you think you are?" or "What are you thinking? You can't do that." What are some tips and tricks you use to combat your own 'stinking thinking'?

Hey, what do you mean? I don't fail! Joking aside, of course there are things that you fail at. Things in life you don't do. One of the hardest parts of aging, even as healthy as I am, at some point you begin to realize that you just can't do what you used to do. I don't mean just physically. No matter what it is, there is a sense that you have to dumb down. That's a reality I face often. My balance, for example, is not as good as it used to be. Interestingly, my balance is better if I am running than if I am walking. I know that sounds counter intuitive.

Getting used to where you are in life, as opposed to where you used to be in life, is an important part of the aging process. It's a bit like the six-year-old who says, "I'm going to be president of the United States when I grow up." Then a bit later he says, "I'm going to be vice president." Then he says, "I'm going to be a senator." Then maybe a congressman. At some point, if none of those things have happened, we have to adjust our expectations and come to grips with our current reality. Part of the aging process is learning how to live with limitations, disappointments, and the current reality.

I am scared of getting injured. I'm scared of

falling and breaking a leg. I'm scared of any injury which might stop me from doing what I am doing. I got away from that sedentary lifestyle when I was 32. To go back to that would be extremely difficult for me.

Physical activity has a very positive effect on my mental state. My wife died several years ago; exercise has really helped me cope with the loss. I live in a retirement community with great facilities and opportunities for social connection. I have three children, six grandchildren, two great-grandchildren who live close by. I am very fortunate in terms of relationships and a sense of community. Thankfully, all these things combined keep my thoughts pretty positive.

Injuries & illness – have you had any major setbacks health-wise? How do you cope with injuries? Do you do anything to avoid injuries? What tips do you have for healing and recovery?

When you get to be my age, your body has been through a lot. I ran my last marathon with a compression fracture of the twelfth vertebrae and pneumonia. I remember having pneumonia years ago. It put me out of commission for six months. Thankfully, this latest bout was a much milder case. I just did what I had to do to take care of myself.

The compression fracture is different. A compression fracture is a fracture in your vertebrae that is caused by crushing rather than breaking. Typically, this happens to older people. They'll go to sit down, miss the chair, and their butt hits the ground. That's how the vertebrae get compressed. That's something I just live with.

When I was in my 70s, I slipped on sand while I was running in Gettysburg, Pennsylvania. I went down hard. People rushed over to help me. As I fell, one side of my body broke my fall. I had nasty abrasions on my leg and arm. I ended up going to the emergency room. They bandaged me up and off I went.

Oh, I've also been bitten by a rattlesnake while out running. I remember coming back in the house and telling my wife, "I just got bitten by a rattlesnake. Will you take me to the emergency room?" I thought she was going to die right then and there. You should have seen the look on her face.

She asked, "How did you know it was a rattlesnake?" I said, "It rattled!" Needless to say, we quickly headed off to the emergency room. They kept me overnight and ran some tests. I learned that 50% of all rattlesnake bites are harmless. When they bite, although their teeth go into the skin, they don't always inject poison. Let me tell you, poison or no poison, a rattlesnake bite hurts like the devil.

I'd love to hear about what inspires you... Who are your role models? How do you stay motivated?

My role models are all dead! Joking aside; it's hard to say. In terms of running, no one comes to mind. In terms of my career, I was interested in achieving and creating a different life for myself. I was born in the depths of the Depression. As a family, we were as poor as poor could be. I wasn't disinterested in making money; however, I was more interested in achieving and having a decent life.

Jeff Galloway's and Jim Fixx's books have helped with motivation. They helped me get from taking those first painful steps around the block to thinking, "Well, why not run a marathon?" Following those guys is probably what got me started and what's kept me going.

Another motivator was turning 70. When I got to 70, I realized that if I wanted to stay in shape, I would have to run two marathons a year. With 52 weeks in a year. It takes about 26 weeks to get in shape to run a marathon. Once one is done, then you have another 26 weeks to get ready for the next marathon. With a commitment of two marathons a year, you never get out of shape. I know that once I'm signed up, I am committed. No excuses.

As you reflect on your accomplishments, what are one or two things that stand out the most for you?

That's a tough question. I have been running for almost 50 years. The Boston Strong Marathon stands out in my mind. This was the marathon the year after the tragic bombing during the 2013 Boston Marathon. There was this incredible sense of pride and commitment. We were not going to let these terrorists interrupt this incredible Patriots' Day celebration. The Boston Marathon is an iconic race, the oldest marathon on the planet. The marathon has been held annually since 1897. Running the Boston Marathon, the year after the bombings, was one of those things I had to do. So, at 80 years old, I did it – in the slowest time humanly possible – but I did it!

The Boston Marathon also stands out to me for other reasons. Up until four or five years ago, Boston was the only marathon in the world for which you had to qualify. You have to qualify by running on a certified course to qualify in your age category. When I was running in my 50s and 60s, I knew I wasn't fast enough to qualify. Once I turned 70 years old, I suddenly realized, "My God, I'm eligible. I can get in!" For me, qualifying for the Boston Marathon felt like a huge accomplishment.

The New York Marathon is a bit different, because they use a lottery system for their entrants. If you have applied three times in succession and didn't get in on the first attempts, you are automatically eligible on the fourth try. I have run the New York Marathon several times. I love that race because of the diversity, the neighborhoods. And the crowds are phenomenal. The Philadelphia Marathon is another great race for runners and spectators. That race is an out-and-back combination, which starts and ends at the famed Rocky statue.

I have also run in lots of foreign countries – 32 to be exact. Not marathons, but just for fun, while traveling. I ran in Johannesburg, South Africa, when Mandela was in prison. That was an eye-opening experience, to see Apartheid first-hand. I have experienced many European cities from a runner's perspective. I've also run in Beijing, China. That was quite an experience. Of course, Beijing is the capital of China. Partly due to a rapidly growing economy the city is known for severe traffic congestion, pollution, and lack of regard for the safety of pedestrians. Our translator actually told us, "Stop signs, red lights, and those sorts of things, are just suggestions."

Another experience that stands out in my mind is Bogota, Columbia. While working for the U.S. Department of Education I attended a conference in Bogota. The attendees included an array of educators and chief school officers from North, South, and Central America.

The conference center was high up in the mountains, probably an elevation of 10,000 feet. Anyway, I would go out for my daily run. I remember people looking at me like I was a real nut case – they were probably right.

I was there because the U.S. Ambassador to Columbia, Diego Cortes Asencio, had been kidnapped, along with 12 other diplomats, by a rogue guerrilla group. The president, Jimmy Carter, felt it was too dangerous to send a high ranking official, so he decided to send me. At the time, I was the newly appointed assistant secretary in the Department of Education. At the Department we joked that I was the most expendable! Anyway, I went down there and attended those meetings. I ran regardless; and thankfully I wasn't kidnapped. So, yes. With 50 years of running, I've seen a lot and had some unique experiences.

If you were to coach a friend, in a similar age range, who was thinking about trying a new sport or wanted to get out there to start moving, what would you tell them?

Based on my experience, motivation is the key. You simply can't motivate somebody who's not interested in changing. Find something that's really going to motivate you. In my case, my motivation came from being a heavy smoker. I started smoking long before the first Surgeon General's report was published. I was also 50 pounds overweight, sitting on the couch waiting for a heart attack. Staring into the eyes of an early death was my motivation!

No joke, colleagues of mine were dying of heart attacks on a regular basis. People thought the cause was over exertion – running to catch that bus or shoveling snow. We now know the cause of death was more likely an unhealthy, sedentary lifestyle. The notion finally settled into my brain that cardiovascular exercise was good for me and smoking was bad. It was that realization that got me motivated. From that point, I was committed to change.

In all honesty, it took me another 10 years to completely quit smoking. I think some of us are more prone to addiction that others. Nicotine affects some of us worse than others, and I am extremely thankful to be free from it. I've had good friends, very intelligent people, who tried and tried to quit. One of them ended up on oxygen. She would literally disconnect her oxygen tank to go out on the deck and smoke a cigarette. That's a powerful addiction.

Running is my mood stabilizer. Running gets oxygen to my brain and my body. At this stage in my life, it's not so much about running this or running that. I simply enjoy getting those shoes on and heading outside.

If you had the one piece of sage advice to share with the world what would it be?

That's a tough question. If the person were already a runner, I'd say listen to your body and don't overdo it. Avoid overuse and self-induced injuries. If you are a new runner or a runner who wants to increase his or her distance, I would recommend Jeff Galloway's program.

I think I have been able to run pretty consistently without any major injuries, because I trust my body to guide me. If I start to notice pain in my calf, knee, or hip when running, I take note mentally. If the pain subsides, then comes back a little stronger, then subsides, then comes back again, I stop running. I know the pain is a warning sign indicating a problem. Pain is like the check-engine light coming on in your car. If the pain goes away, then the issue has probably worked itself out. I have never had any ankle, knee, hip injuries, and I've been running for the best part of 50 years.

Any final thoughts or reflections?

When I think about where I came from, all the incredible opportunities I've had, and the joy running has brought to my life, I feel very, very fortunate.

———

SISTER MADONNA BUDER

Also known as the Iron Nun. Who at 87 years old
is a world champion triathlete.

*"Be the best you, you can be in the present
moment."*

– Sister Madonna Buder

I WAS NOT AWARE of Sister Madonna's existence, let
alone her accolades until a friend told me about "a
nun who a runs triathlons." I was hoping to find a
later-in-life female triathlete to complete the book.
Yet again, a Google search led me to her door.

In October 1953 Madonna Buder dedicated her
life to Christ. Along with her duties as a Sister she
had a talent for running. At the age of 52 Sister
Madonna ran her first marathon in a time of three
hours and 29 minutes. Fast enough to qualify for the
Boston Marathon. With the blessing of the Priest she
was given permission to run the Boston Marathon
and raise money for multiple sclerosis. That was
the beginning of a lifetime of incredible athletic
endeavors.

As I mentioned in the introduction, I was
surprised that an athlete of this caliber agreed to an
interview. I remember feeling nervous as I prepped

for our phone conversation. Our call was scheduled for early one beautiful Sunday morning in July. I'm not sure if it was the fact that she was a nun or a world renowned athlete. Regardless, I had this feeling in my gut that said, "This is important; don't screw it up."

Sister Madonna answered the phone. At 87 years old, she was as sharp as a tack. No messing around. She jumped straight into the conversation asking me about my methods, experience as a writer, and details about my publisher. I responded like a bumbling buffoon. All tongue tied with ums and ahs. Honestly, it was painful. Then when I managed to spit out that, in fact, I was self-publishing and that this was my first book project, there was a bit too much silence. For a moment I thought the conversation was dead in the water.

Of course, Sister Madonna was nothing but gracious. We found a commonality as we shared stories about marathon swimmers. Specifically, Sister Madonna shared more about how inspirational Diana Nyad's story was about her lifetime dream of swimming from Cuba to Florida. After five attempts Diana completed the swim. She was 62 years old.

Sister Madonna seamlessly steered the conversation toward my first question about 'must read' books. Pretty soon, with all her wonderful stories, laughter, and infectious energy we soon fell into a comfortable flow.

By the end of the hour I was feeling comfortable enough to express how nervous I felt going into the conversation. Sister Madonna took the time to inquire as to why I felt that way. On reflection, I was able to express that something deeper drew me to this conversation. I felt the conversation was important. Meaningful. Inspirational.

Ultimately, I felt honored and grateful to be given the opportunity to talk to this remarkable woman who has selflessly done so much and inspired so many. With heartfelt thanks...

Sister Madonna

What is your favorite quote or saying?

"God, help me do my best, and you do the rest."

I conceived this saying when I was recovering from a torn meniscus and didn't want surgery. I remember going home and saying, "God, help me do my best, and you do the rest." It just had a catchy rhythm and rhyme to it. I can stand by it anytime. It's good for any situation, not just physical, but any situation you meet in life where you need God's assistance. Of course, you still have to do your best, but you can also invite God to do the rest. That's a winning team!

Can you think of a book that stands out in your mind as an influential 'must read'?

Have you ever read *Find a Way* by Diana Nyad? This is a remarkable story, a must-read if you have a chance. Diana was 27 years old when she first attempted to swim from Cuba to Florida. That swim was fraught with many difficulties. Diana attempted this swim five times. Her fifth attempt was when she was 62 years old. She finally made it! The book and the way she expresses everything is amazing.

Of course, the Bible is a forever must for me. There is another book that is very inspiring. The book is called *On Fire: The 7 Choices to Ignite a Radically Inspired Life* by John O'Leary. It's the story of a nine-year-old boy who was burned all over his body and not expected to live. He survived. He's married and has children. John shares his story and does podcast interviews – very inspiring.

Please share a bit about your background. How did you get interested in this sport, and what were some of your first steps?

I got introduced to triathlons via running. It all started on the Oregon coast where the Sisters and I were attending a conference with a priest. He arrived the evening before, and we had the opportunity to sit around the table and have some informal discussion. As we talked, the priest started expounding about the benefits of running. I thought, "Well, that's kind of stupid." I thought running was just a silly fad. This was in 1977. Of course, being a

Sister removed from the greater populace, I didn't know anything about this running fad.

As a kid, I was very active and always outdoors. I love the sun. When I was two, I had my first experience with swimming. While on vacation near Lake Michigan, my father took me out on the pier. I guess I wriggled free and took my first plunge. He quickly dove in and grabbed me. Expecting sobbing and gasping, there was no fear. I was giggling, and apparently quite delighted with myself.

I have always been attracted to outdoor activities. During my school years, I remember longing to be outside playing Kick the Can, Cops and Robbers, or just running around. In my teens, my passion for horses grew and I became an accomplished equestrian. College came and went. By the time I was 26, I had worked and taken my final vows. I dedicated my life to God and became a member of the Sisters of the Good Shepherd.

Running did not enter my life until I was 48 years old. During a retreat, Father John Topel talked to our group about the benefits of running. He shared emerging research about how running can harmonize body and soul and help with addictions, depression, stress, and diabetes. Although I valued physical activity, now, as an adult, I just couldn't see myself getting out there to run for no good reason; I needed a goal. The Father suggested, "Well, you know what? Out there on the beach, there are two eddies. Go and run between them without getting wet."

Thinking about what the priest said about running harmonizing the mind, body, and soul caught my attention. Later that evening, after rummaging through a pile of donated clothes, I pulled out a pair of shorts and an old pair of running shoes and set out to run between the eddies. I headed down to the beach in the dark and started running. It felt so good.

After my run, I came in through the side door, and who was there but Father Topel. He inquired, "Oh, where have you been?" I replied, "Out doing what you said."

Surprised, he asked, "Well, how far did you go?"

"Between the two eddies," I replied.

"How long did it take you?" he asked.

"Oh, about five minutes or so," I replied.

He asked how often I stopped. I told him I hadn't stopped. He asked if I had any idea how far that was. I knew it was about half a mile because I used to walk it all the time. The priest seemed impressed. He said, "Well, you can't stop now. You've got to do this for at least five weeks before you get the runner's high."

I was confused, thinking you were supposed to get that in prayer. I didn't realize that was what running was all about. To this day, even after all the triathlons and running events, do I know what the runner's high is? I don't think so. I sure know what the lows are. At the time, I had no idea where this running thing would take me. Like many things in my life, I just stepped out in faith.

Tell me about some of the joys, challenges, and milestones along the way.

One of biggest challenges that stands out in my memory is from 2006. A week before the Ironman event in Hawaii, a big earthquake hit. This never happens. They get storms and hurricanes, but an earthquake is very unusual. The earthquake affected a tiny portion of the bike course. The race director assessed the damage as minimal, and the message was "Come on down."

When I got there, it wasn't the typical Hawaiian atmosphere. The weather was overcast and a lot cooler than usual. The airport was stacked full of bikes, equipment, and passengers scrambling for flights. It was bananas. After navigating the airport and the traffic, I finally arrived at the place I was staying and settled in for the night. In the early hours of the morning, I was woken by a shaking sensation. It felt like someone was rattling a cage. I quickly realized, "Uh oh, we're getting aftershocks." These aftershocks were a full week after the first earthquake.

The aftershocks continued throughout the morning of the race. Of course, the swim is the first part of the course. After swimming for a while, I noticed I was not seeing the landmarks one would expect to see. My thoughts pondered, "Hmm, I've been swimming for a while. I don't think I'm making any progress."

Somehow the earthquake seemed to be stirring up a hurricane, making the current much stronger than usual. This, of course, made the swim much longer and harder than it normally would be. The conditions added at least 20 minutes to my time based on my previous performance. I remember thinking to myself, "Well, this looks like it's going to be a long day."

With the swim behind me, it was time for the bike portion of the race. At about halfway through the bike course, the rain started. The heavy rain was compounded by strong winds creating driving rain blasting full force into my face. The conditions were so bad I was forced to shut my eyes. This was my first experience of racing a bike with my eyes closed. I'm thinking to myself, "Well, my sunglasses don't have windshield wipers, so the only thing I can do is just shut my eyes and hope for the best." Of course, that slowed the bike portion of the race down considerably. Then we came to the run. I heard this little 'put, put, put' behind me, and I thought, "Uh oh, this means I must be the last runner." Sure enough, the man on the moped came up and said, "You're nine minutes down." First, I thought, "What in the world is he talking about?" Then I realized he's trying to tell me that I'm nine minutes away from making the cutoff time of 17 hours. "Well," I said to myself, "I'd better pick up the pace."

Low and behold, it starts to pour with rain again. People dashed for shelter, even the guy on the moped. There I am, out there, ankle deep in water with this little voice saying to me, "If you keep running, you could fall. And you're so weak. If you can't get up, you won't make it."

I thought, "OK, I won't run. I'll just shuffle." I headed for the opposite side of the road where there was a sidewalk. I was still on the course, but I was hoping to get better leverage. Just as I started to step up onto the curb, I immediately crashed. With the torrential rain, I couldn't see the curb. I came crashing down on my knee.

Was I bleeding? Did I break something? I had no idea how bad the fall was. Out of nowhere, this couple appeared, and they started helping me up. I don't know who they were or where they came from. I was so dazed. I don't think I even said thank you. Once I was back on my feet, I continued running. Pretty soon, I got to the aid station at the halfway point. I knew my body needed some nourishment. I was hoping for some hot chicken soup.

I made two mistakes. The first mistake was sitting down. My second mistake was eating the lukewarm chicken soup. You know what lukewarm does to your stomach? Then I spied a Parker House roll. I thought eating that would help absorb some of the liquid sloshing around down there in my stomach. The roll didn't help either. I sat down to rest for a moment. Before I knew it, one of the volunteers at the aid station started to massage my neck and back. By that point, the last thing I wanted to do was get back on my feet. From way back inside my head, I remember this little voice saying, "Nobody's going to finish this race for you. You'd better get up and do it now!"

So, obediently I got up and made my way back down to the course. The next section was the worst portion of the course. It was very dark. With no lights, and very difficult to see where you are going. As I came out of that area, I know there's about two miles down and two miles back up to the main road. I remember giving myself a pep talk. "All right, I've got six miles left to go. Maybe, just maybe, I can do this."

By that time, another guy on his moped whizzed by. He was an announcer, someone I recognized from previous races I had been in. What I didn't know was that he was radioing back to the people at the finish line telling them where Sister Madonna was and whether she was going to make it or not because of all the nip and tuck. Of course, I didn't know any of this.

Then, out of nowhere, four people came out of the dark and headed across the road toward me.

"May we run with you?" they asked. I replied, "Can't you see I'm not running?" Undeterred they replied, "Well, can we escort you?" I said OK. As a gesture of support, they offered to tell me a story – a classic means of distraction. By that point, I was completely depleted of any brain power. I mumbled, "Yes, please…"

I recognized that two of the people were native Hawaiians. One was wearing thongs [flip flops], the other was barefoot. The other two people were a married couple wearing running shoes. I remember thinking, "There's no way these guys are going to make it for six miles with no shoes." I don't care what we're doing, walking or crawling, they're never going to make it.

At some point, the guys without shoes peeled out. The couple stayed with me until the last mile and a quarter, which is a downhill section. The couple firmly instructed, "Now, don't stop running when you get to the bottom, just keep going." My usual MO for this course is to make a beeline down the hill, turn the corner, and then walk from exhaustion. I thought, "How can they possibly know this? How do they know I usually do this?" The whole thing was uncanny.

I took their advice. I got to the bottom of the hill. It took me all I had to keep running, but I kept going. Then, once again, this little voice from deep inside: "What you are doing is unreal. It's like reality is being superimposed on unreality." Instinctively, I knew it would take a miracle to beat the 17-hour cutoff time. Regardless, I pleaded for a sign to indicate my recently deceased nephew was at peace and in the right place.

Then, in the dark, I felt this presence behind my right shoulder. I don't know how to best describe it, but this presence stayed by my side until I turned the corner to head down the last stretch toward the finish line. By this point, crowds of people had gathered. Traditionally, spectators put their hands out to give high fives to give runners encouragement. Generally, I would reciprocate. But this time, that little voice spoke again, loud and clear: "Don't touch anybody. If you do, you could stagger back. It could cost you seconds, which you can't spare." "Oh, OK," I unquestioningly obeyed. On I go through the cheering crowds getting closer and closer to the finish line.

For some ungodly reason, this year, instead of a flat, straight-through run to the finish line, the race organizers had decided to build a ramp. Competitors had to run up the ramp to reach the finish line. That took every last ounce of strength I had in me. When I got to the top, I bent over and started dry heaving. Of course, there were cameramen, reporters, and crowds of people all around. All I could think was, "What a great picture this is. Me with the dry heaves."

After gathering myself a bit, I was able to stand up. I looked at the time; it was absolutely unreal. The clock read 16 hours, 59 minutes and 3 seconds. The announcer and the crowds were going crazy.

The same exuberant announcer had attended the pre-race party for the 60-plus competitors. Over the years, he got to know me fairly well. I remember asking him if he could report on the different genders as they crossed the finish line. "You know, it would be great if you could you announce male or female. Could you at least say, 'Iron Woman'?" I had asked.

The announcer waffled a bit saying something about having to "discuss that with the higher-ups." I'm not sure if he ever had those discussions. Regardless, he got so excited about my finish. Right over the speaker, loud and clear, I heard, "Iron Woman, you made it! You made it!" The announcer was bouncing up and down, unable to contain himself.

I remember him interviewing me at the finish line. I responded to one of his questions by saying, "This is a miracle which I attribute to my deceased nephew." I dedicated this race to my nephew who died unexpectedly the previous month. Nobody knew what caused his death. The coroners were in the midst of an autopsy, which, at this point, hadn't revealed any clues. The announcer, delirious with delight shouted, "Yep, he's at peace and in the right place!" That's a race which will stick with me forever.

Thinking about food as fuel, what have you tried diet-wise? What has been helpful? Are there any supplements you swear by? Do you have any must-have foods when training or competing? What is a treat in your world?

I do take herbs and vitamins. Food-wise, I usually eat raw foods, mostly vegetables and fruit. Raw food is where you get the real vitamins. I also eat chicken and fish now and again. Occasionally, if I'm out to dinner, I'll go for the beef, but other than that, my diet is very simple. Plus, I cut down on preparation time by eating everything raw.

It's amazing how my tastes have changed through the years. I used to be a big Pepsi fan. None of the diet stuff; for some reason, I just preferred full sugar Pepsi over Coke. Now, I don't drink any soda. I also used to be addicted to peanut M&Ms, and I don't eat those anymore either. I am missing five teeth. I have a partial tooth for two of them. At this point in my life, I have to eat food that doesn't take too much crunching or my gums get sore.

How did you begin to build your fitness? What were some of your early steps? And how did you know you were starting to form a habit?

I think it was after I did my first Ironman. I remember that race like it was yesterday. Back then, I was not a strong swimmer. I really had no clue about what I was doing. That particular year was the year the race organizers decided to make the swim cutoff time at an hour and 15 minutes. As I got closer to the pier, I remember thinking, "Oh my God, the scenery is not changing down below me. How am I ever going to get to the pier?" At that point, it was clear that I wasn't going to make the swim cutoff time.

Well, I finally made it to the shore. As people were dragging me to my feet, I realized I was four minutes too late. This meant I couldn't go on to compete in the rest of the race. As an aside, had the cutoff time been what it is today, I would have made it. Regardless, I headed back to where I was staying and washed my hair, feeling like Nellie from the musical *South Pacific* – "I'm going to wash this [race] right out of my hair..." Then I headed back out to the racecourse.

I retrieved my bike out of transition, something you could never do today. I went back out on the course, two hours behind the pack. I knew I wouldn't be interfering with anybody's race. I was just observing and encouraging people who were coming on the course in the opposite direction. I hadn't planned this. Heading back out on the course was an impulsive decision.

I was hungry and thirsty after the swim; somehow it didn't occur to me to bring a water bottle or any food. I remember feeling depleted and thinking, "Now what I have done?" No sooner than I had that thought, a young man working at the aid station I was passing saw me and came running over with a banana. I recall thinking, "Well, thank you, Lord, I will accept that."

I rode on and got as far as I could before climbing up the long 14-mile stretch to the turnaround point. I saw this lone Japanese man heading down toward me. There was no one else around him. I thought, "You know what? There's no sense in me going up there. I don't even know if the aid station is open." I noticed a staff car perched on the side of the mountain reporting back to the finish line. Making eye contact, I yelled, "Do you think the aid station is open up there?" "Err, we doubt it," they chimed, confirming my thoughts.

At this point, I decided to turn around and try to catch up with the Japanese guy and give him some encouragement. I was exhausted, hot, and very hungry. The staff wagon, finishing their duties, headed down the mountain toward me. They stopped. "Would you like a lift? Maybe something to eat or drink?" they offered. With immense gratitude I gasped, "Yes." They inquired, "What would you like?" And I said, "All three please."

I got in the car as they loaded my bike into the back. After I had something to drink, we got to chatting. Knowing I was a nun, they asked if I knew there was a priest out there. Apparently, there was an Episcopalian priest who was also racing. They wondered if he was a Catholic priest or maybe I knew him. "Look, look. There he is now," they pointed.

As we passed him, I got his race number. I said, "You can let me off here." They stopped the car, unloaded my bike, and let me out. They offered to hold my bike for me. I said, "No, no. I can get on. Uh oh, there he goes," I said, and hurried to get my bike. "It's all right," they said. "You'll catch him on the hill." Sure enough, that's exactly what happened.

As I caught up to the priest I said, "Padre, there's a Japanese man in front of you, if you hurry up, you're going to catch him." Then I rode ahead, up to the Japanese guy, and said, "You know what? There's somebody behind you who's the last runner, so you better hurry up."

I kept seesawing, back and forth between the two racers, encouraging them to step it up. The pastor was a competitor from the previous year. He had missed the final cutoff time at the finish; he was back trying again this year. At that time, the course had a vicious hill climb about a mile and a half before the transition from the bike section of the race to the run section – the final leg before the finish line. Knowing the course, I remember thinking, "OK, this Padre is not going to make it up that hill."

I rode to the top of the hill and got off my bike. I waited and waited, and sure enough, there he was, walking his bike up the hill. As soon as he got back on his bike, I said, "All right. You have to go for broke. You have no time left!" He got back on his bike and rode that last bit.

By the time the Padre started out on the run, it was getting dark. With no light, I was not visible on the bike. It was at that point when I realized, "Oh my God, it's dark. I've got to get myself back into town." I knew there would be children all over the place, running back and forth. I knew it would not be safe to follow and encourage him anymore.

The Padre had a little inspirational note taped on the handlebars of his bike. It read, "Go for God." As I left him, I yelled, "OK, Padre, you are on your own. Go for God!"

The next morning, I got up and went to check on the results. The Padre finished his race with two minutes to spare! It was then when I knew that running and triathlons had become an integral part of my life. The next year, I went back and finished the race. Since that time, I have successfully completed the Hawaiian Ironman triathlon at least 22 times. Since that first attempt, I have also completed the Canadian Ironman 22 or 23 times. All in all, I've probably completed close to 45 Ironman or Iron *Woman* races.

Do you have any morning or evening routines?
Actually, I don't; every day is different.

Discrimination and/or negativity as an older athlete – do you think this is a thing? Have you personally experienced it? How did you deal with it? What would you tell others?

Discrimination or negativity has not been an issue for me. When I reached 60, I thought, I'm finished with this. There's no more reason to go on. Then when I got to 70, I said, OK, doing this isn't going to mean anything to anybody. But I continued anyway. Now in my 80s, I'm suddenly an inspiration for so many people. I don't know why except for the fact that I'm old.

Also, I don't allow trivialities to get in my way. People have been encouraging. When you're running, usually you have your number on the back of your calf. I often get younger triathletes passing me on the run, yelling, "I want to be like you when I grow up." I yell back, "Then don't grow up!"

I do think our culture regarding age has changed through the years. Europeans and Asians tend to revere age. Here in the U.S., we try to knock each other out instead. I see those limiting views are beginning to shift and change. I attribute this shift to people like me – older athletes who are out there showing people what can be done. Keep on keeping on!

We all have thoughts that can be negative: fears, doubts, that critical voice that might say, "Who do you think you are?" or "What are you thinking? You can't do that." What are some tips and tricks you use to combat your own 'stinking thinking'?

I remember one Canadian Ironman in particular. I had eight miles to go over a course that took us out along a river. There were no streetlights. It was dark, and the footing was kind of touchy. I was feeling nauseous and tired. That little voice from the left side inside my head said, "If somebody comes to pick you up, just let them do it. You're finished." Then, another voice on the right side of my head countered, "No, don't give up. Just keep trying." So, while the two voices were battling away with each other, I decided, "No, I'm going to keep on plugging away," which I did against all odds. Sometimes the battle is within yourself and you just have to recognize it and push through.

Injuries & illness – have you had any major setbacks health-wise? How do you cope with injuries? Do you do anything to avoid injuries? What tips do you have for healing and recovery?

I never got sick or had any major mishaps when I was young. It seems I had to wait until I was in my second childhood before I had to deal with injuries because of my occupation. At this point in my life, I don't think there's a part of my body that hasn't been injured. I recall getting one injury during training: a broken hip, I think. Honestly, I can't keep track of them all.

My most recent injury was in 2014. I experienced three major setbacks in a 16-month period. One of those injuries was a torn meniscus. I managed to squeeze in a triathlon on either side of that injury. The doctors are always amazed once they realize my age. They'll say, "Now, you know it's going to take 10 weeks to heal." With the torn meniscus, I said, "No, I can't afford that amount of time. I have a race coming up in five weeks." So, I did whatever I could to speed my recovery.

I believe that when you are in the hospital having surgery and you're lying still in bed, sleep is beneficial. However, circulation is also necessary. Since I live alone, and I'm graced with long arms, I can reach everything I need in my little apartment. I can do everything for myself without any assistance. This keeps my body circulating and speeds the healing and recovery process. After the torn meniscus, I had one week to get on the bike before the race. I was able to complete that triathlon with little to no training.

I'd love to hear about what inspires you... Who are your role models? How do you stay motivated?

Well, I must admit that even running, which used to be my forte – after all, that's how I entered triathlons was through running; it's not enjoyable to me. Of the three sports, running is the hardest thing for me right now. I have to push my body to run. All

I can say is that it's become a discipline. I have to discipline myself. It's not through enjoyment. It's through knowing that it's not about me. I keep going for my public's sake.

As you reflect on your accomplishments, what are one or two things that stand out the most for you?

Some things were surprises, like being inducted into the USA Triathlon Hall of Fame in 2013. That was a complete surprise. I got that news when I was recovering from an injury. Somehow, I had to make it up on the stage and hug the person that was presenting me with the award.

Recently, I received an award here in Spokane from the Spokane Sports Commission, which I didn't know existed. They awarded me as an honorary member and asked me to give a little talk. I just take it all in my stride.

Sometimes it's easy to fret and worry about what you have to do, the things that lie in front of you. I constantly remind myself that worrying and fretting are useless because what I see as happening in the future might not be at all what happens when the future actually gets to be the present moment.

I remember my grandmother, who was a very insightful person, giving me a bit of advice. I was nine years old, sitting at the top of the staircase with my head in my hands, staring in front of me pondering. As my grandmother came in the front door, she looked up toward the banister and saw me. She said, "Darling, what's the matter?" I replied, "Well, I'm just wondering what I should do when I grow up." I now realize that she could have laughed, but she didn't. Instead, she looked straight at me and said, "Well, darling, let's look at it this way. The past is dead and gone, never to return. The future is not the future until it gets here. All you are responsible for is living in the present moment, and what you do in the present moment will lead you into the future."

That made so much sense to me. Right then and there, her words just took the load off my shoulders immediately. Now, when I do service work in jail, I share this story. As you can imagine, there's a lot of worry going on in jail. Worry happens because we get stuck and rutted in the future where we don't belong. The future is up to God. What we do in the present moment is up to us. My advice: be the best you can be in the present moment.

If you were to coach a friend, in a similar age range, who was thinking about trying a new sport or wanted to get out there to start moving, what would you tell them?

You know, I don't tell anybody anything. For instance, recently there was a couple from a company in California who is interested in doing a documentary about religion and sports. They were here for four days following me around, documenting whatever I did. During that time, I did a little run for Father's Day.

The two of them were totally impressed. Although they had been acquainted with activity, neither of them was active on a regular basis. After shadowing me for a couple of days, on their own accord, they decided to start an exercise practice and stick to it. Now they're off, as busy as they are, going around the country, stalking other people, and making time for their own exercise routine. Doing by example is so much more powerful than words.

If you had the one piece of sage advice to share with the world what would it be?

Trust. Just trust. The Bible is full of examples of how people were able to overcome all kinds of things by trusting in their supreme maker. In my opinion, we do not refer to Him, or Her, often enough. It sets us back when we think we can do everything by ourselves. When we invite our maker to suggest, to be in control, we have a much easier life than thinking we can control everything by ourselves. We need to trust in the Father. Someone who is wiser than us. Adopting a little humility is very, very necessary to live by faith and in trust.

Any final thoughts or reflections?

For the longest time, I felt that I needed to write a sequel to my book, *The Grace to Race*, and call it

The Race to Grace, but I haven't had the time. At one point, when I was ready to give up the Ironman distance, because of what happened in my last attempt, I figured that that would be the time. Instead, everything started to pick up again and life seems busier than ever. I don't know, maybe I'll have to be 100 before I have the time to get that second book done. Enjoy life as you live it.

―――――

LIMITING BELIEFS
AND MOTIVATION

"Don't let yesterday take up too much of today."
– Will Rogers

IT TAKES A LOT to get-up, dressed, and out of the house to the gym, trail head, or track; to go for that run, hike, or bike ride. When problem solving and coaching through the 'whys' as in, "Why the heck am I having such a difficult time with this?" or "Why can't I get off the couch?" people often point to motivation, or the lack there of, as the culprit.

In my practice, as a mental health professional, I help people create lifestyles that include sustainable wellness and performance, along with a whole list of other stuff. Honestly, if I had a dollar for every time I've heard, "I just can't get motivated," well...

In my opinion, trying to figure out motivation strategies before, what I call, the deeper limiting beliefs have been examined is a concern. It's like having a vintage sports car that's been sitting in the garage. It's a beautiful day. You decide to take it for a spin. Great! There's a bit of gas in the tank;

enough to get you a few miles. You head out – life is good! Suddenly, clunckty, clunk, clunk – the car grinds to a halt. Crap. You get out, look under the hood, and realize it's not the gas; other vital fluids have been ignored.

When trying to ignite motivation, examining our thoughts seems like a logical place to start – "Hmm, let's see, what are my thoughts telling me?" Once we *think* (pun intended) we have figured the thoughts out, then, in an attempt to increase motivation we start brain-storming. We create action plans, set goals, and make to-do lists. Again, we use that *thinking* part of our brain to come up with all the things we could do. We get creative. We lay our gym clothes out the night before. We set the alarm clock to get-up half an hour earlier. We plaster our worlds with affirmations (I am particularly good at that one...). Of course, this is all great. However, it's not getting at the disconnect under the hood.

OK, enough with the metaphors. Let me clarify. When I talk about 'under the hood stuff', I am referring to our deeper processes – what I call the *back-brain* stuff. When we think we are using our frontal cortex (front-brain). Our deeper felt senses – feelings, intuitions, etc. come from deep inside our brain (back-brain). At this juncture, it's important to note that the brain, motivation, and how it all works is still very much a mystery. Clearly, the above is an oversimplification of highly complex processes.

Like I said, thoughts are great. However, when someone's really stuck, I want to go deeper. I want to dig into that back-brain stuff. I want to ferret out the core beliefs that are lurking quietly beneath the surface; somewhere in that back-brain there's probably a limiting belief creating a barrier. In an attempt to take lofty biopsychosocial concepts about how our beliefs are formed and make time tested theories digestible, here's how I break it down.

Straight out of the shoot we basically land in a petri dish. Within that *dish* we have systems. Here are some of the common systems: family (close and extended), friends, school, sports, religions (whatever flavor that might be), and community.

This is where the petri dish analogy comes in. As new little humans, we *all* land in our personal petri dish which is adorned with systems. Mammals, especially humans, spend a good portion of our lives swimming around in that dish soaking-up everything those powerful systems have to offer. We take it all in – the good, the bad, and the ugly – it's unavoidable.

Now fast-forward to adulthood. Yes, we grow up and head out into the world. We make all sorts of smart, logical, front brain decisions. Yet, we are also very capable of making decisions that are not so great. If it were simply our thoughts running the show, I contend that we would be much better at using that highly logical thinking part of our brain, which – logically (again, pun intended) – would lead to super logical behavior.

If it were that easy, wouldn't we all have our gym bags neatly packed by the door ready for the chime of that early morning alarm bell? Wouldn't it be effortless to spring out of bed just because our thoughts commanded it? Wouldn't we all be fit and healthy simply because we 'know' it's good for us? I can tell you, at least in my experience, this is generally not the case.

The point I am trying to make is that somewhere along the way we have *all* soaked up limiting beliefs that are unhelpful. In doing my own work around the topic of motivation I realized that I had a sneaky limiting belief around 'being lazy'. Once I was able to put this deeper sense, or feeling, into words I was able to work with it.

When I fact-check myself I am clearly not lazy. I run, hike, write, have two jobs, take care of a home, run a business, etc. That 'belief' was clearly old back-brain stuff coming up. It's also a fact that I didn't come out of the shoot thinking "I'm lazy." Right then, I knew this was petri dish stuff, which interestingly provided some relief – OK, I thought, "I'm not inherently lazy; that's old back-brain stuff I can work through. I don't have to buy into that anymore. Cool!"

With a bit more digging I was able to trace the origins of this unhelpful belief to my early teens.

Somewhere, during that glorious period when I was sleeping until noon, obnoxious, and expected the world to revolve around me – I connected with the sense of soaking up messaging around 'you're so lazy.' The originating sources were likely my family system around chores (particularly cleaning my room) and the school system – stuff around 'not trying hard enough' – which I, in my adolescent brain, internalized as 'being lazy' – is the best I could get to.

"What!" I hear you saying. "That was literally 40 years ago; this is now. Get over yourself already." Alright, slow down a moment... Once I was able to get to the root of my unhelpful back-brain belief, I was able to retool using the facts from my current life and presto. I'm not saying this limiting belief has been erased from my personal fabric never to be seen again. What I am saying is that now, when I notice the underlying sense of 'I'm lazy' arising, as I consider all the reasons I *shouldn't* head out for that run I planned, I can fact-check myself about the truth of that belief as it pertains to me today. As a result, I am not weighed down by it anymore. Moreover, when it does creep into my thoughts, I can *manage* it without *believing* it's true – a big difference.

If you are finding yourself struggling with motivation or other unhelpful behaviors it might be time to look more deeply under the hood. Here's an exercise you can do if you are interested in some self-discovery. Remember – you CAN change your beliefs.

First...

Get a notepad and pen. Find a quiet space. Go inside and ask yourself:

- What beliefs do I hold that are helpful?

- What beliefs do I hold that are unhelpful?

Note – A helpful belief is something that serves you. It fits with your life today and aligns with your current values. An unhelpful belief is something that hinders you. It doesn't currently serve you, it creates a barrier limiting your progress.

Important: No thinking. No judgement. No "am I doing this right?" – just a free flowing of thoughts, jotting down whatever comes up – again, no judgement needed!

Second...

Once you have a list, it's time to evaluate – this is a front-brain activity. Look at each belief and ask yourself, "Does this belief match with the facts and reality of my life today?" Simply add a yes or no response next to each belief.

> *Note* – This is purely a logical, linear front brain, here and now activity. Put any emotion, critical voice, or judgement aside.

This is where the magic happens – you are actually moving unconscious back-brain stuff into front-brain consciousness. Great work!

Third...

Now you have a list it's time to consider what's helpful and what's unhelpful.

Starting with the unhelpful beliefs begin to work through them one at a time. Here are a couple of inquiries you could make about that unhelpful belief.

Again, go inside and ask yourself:

- Where did this belief come from?
- What is this belief about?
- When did I first hear about this belief?
- How old was I?
- Where was I?
- How *was* this belief helpful?
- Does this belief serve me in my current life?

Note – You might not have answers to all these questions – that's OK. Also, again – no judgement. No blame. Just gentle curiosity.

Fourth...

Once you have a better understanding about this belief and how it developed you can begin to retool the unhelpful belief into something that's a better fit for your life and values today. One way to do this is to re-write your story.

Going back to my personal example of "I'm lazy." Which, as a side note, as I write those words I am actually thinking (front-brain) and believing (back-brain) i.e. feeling it in my emotional system, "That's so ridiculous; I'm not lazy." This, by the way, is exactly the internal response you are looking for.

Re-writing your story

Step 1

Write the story about then. As much as you can remember. Include your age, developmental stage, circumstances, who was around. Once you have a good start on the narrative, check inside for more incidences when this belief came up (past, recent past, present). Throw it all on the page – feel like you have got it all? Good.

Then write the story about how this, now unhelpful belief once served or helped you. Back to my example – being lazy, which as a teen was true at the time. This belief served – or helped me to – avoid things. If I was 'lazy' then expectations were low (at home and school). At home I could isolate myself in my room. At school I could fly under the radar – at least that's what I have figured out thus far.

Step 2

Now it's time to layer in the current details into your story. You guessed it. It's time to fact-check your life as it stands *today*. Shift your perspective to your adult self. In my example today's facts (mentioned above) easily outweigh the unhelpful "I'm lazy" belief. You will likely have a similar experience.

Step 3

Once you have a good inventory. Ask yourself, "Are these current facts really true?" Then ask, "Do I *believe* these current facts are true?" Then inquire, "Is there any here and now evidence to dispute today's facts?" As you do this exercise, stay grounded. Feet firmly on the floor, feeling the ground beneath your feet, your bottom on the chair, and your body rising and falling as you breathe. Sit in this space for a moment or two. Let it all sink in. Repeat this exercise a couple of times a day. Before going to sleep and on waking are particularly powerful times in your day…

Note – These techniques will not magically erase unhelpful beliefs. The old belief will still raise its ugly head now and again. The cool thing is that now you *will* recognize it. Over time you will begin to automatically fact-check yourself creating the ability to put that unhelpful belief aside. This puts you firmly in the driver's seat. Allowing you to put your energy into more helpful here and now beliefs and choices.

Additionally, this exercise provides insight. Personally, I have discovered that the unhelpful "I'm lazy" belief tends to kick-in when I'm tired or feeling rundown. Knowing this, I can retool by checking in with my body. I can figure out what really is going on, then gently remind myself, that I am in fact "tired" not "lazy".

Strengthening new more helpful beliefs

Strengthen, shape, and use your helpful beliefs to reach your goals. Back to my example. Once I realize my body needs rest, I can acknowledge that. The realization that I am dragging because I need a rest creates a very different feeling compared to some back-brain belief about being "lazy" that I soaked up 40 years ago.

With more current, factual information I can now choose to take a 20-minute nap knowing that: one, it's OK, everybody gets tired, and two, from experience I know a nap will give me more energy so I can head out for that run or finish that project.

Furthermore, from a neurological perspective this cycle is highly reinforcing. The brain likes that "I did something right" feeling. As a result, little bursts of feel-good neurotransmitters flood the body increasing the likelihood that I will take action and, in turn, feel more motivated to repeat this cycle again in the future. The more helpful belief cycles are repeated, the stronger the reinforcement becomes; pretty soon the old unhelpful belief is left in the dust.

Although this is fascinating stuff, please know this is a very general overview and is not intended to replace professional help or advice. If, however, you are interested in a deeper dive on the subject I have a book in the works which you might enjoy. Please go to katechampionauthor.com and connect with me to receive updates, information, and publishing news.

———

RESOURCES

"The journey of a thousand miles begins with one step."

– Lao Tzu

THIS CHAPTER IS CRAFTED to help you with the action phase of change. After reading inspirational accounts of ordinary people doing incredible things well into their later years and learning how to change limiting beliefs you might be thinking, "Sure, that's nice; but I could never do anything like that" (probably a limiting belief – just saying). Or, on the other hand, maybe one of the conversations resonated with you, sparking an interest. A curiosity. A wondering: "Hmm, what am I capable of?" "How far could I go?"

This, my friend, is exciting news. When you notice thoughts like that sprouting in your brain it's time to celebrate, cultivate, and nurture – these are the seeds of change!

I realize that starting a new endeavor can seem like a daunting process. However, if you find some seeds sprouting, the next step in the cycle of change is to create some momentum: also known as action.

In this chapter you will find a list of the resources the athletes mention categorized by medium: books, websites, Facebook groups, etc. Where possible I have added descriptions, links, and general blurb to help you streamline the information gathering process. You will also find *suggestions* – these are resources I have personally used or found helpful in my journey.

Lastly, I have added an Appendix with all the races and trails the athletes mention. Where possible I have added the corresponding links.

As I grow as a writer, and a later in life athlete, understanding four things has been invaluable:

- Taking a tiny step is always better than doing nothing.

- Doing a little bit every day will eventually get you there.

- Age is not a limitation.

- It's never too late.

As you review the following, notice what resonates with you. Get curious. Dig around. Play. Use the links to explore. Connect with your imagination; see the possibilities – like a kid in a candy store – wide-eyed with wonder. What do you see yourself doing? Who knows what adventures you will find out there...

Books Mentioned

Annapurna by Maurice Herzog
(memoir/adventure/mountaineer)

This is a memoir about Maurice Herzog, who in the 1950s led an expedition of French climbers to the summit of an 8,075-meter (26,493-foot) Himalayan peak called Annapurna. The expedition chose a route that was unchartered; ascending and descending the mountain using a collection of basic rudimentary maps. Within the pages of *Annapurna* an incredible adventure including vivid accounts of frostbite, snow blindness, and human endurance unfolds.

Born to Run by Christopher McDougall
(memoir/inspirational/ultra-running)

The story of an epic adventure that took McDougall through Mexico's deadly Copper Canyons in search of the famed Tarahumara Indians who, legend has it, have the ability to run hundreds of miles without rest or injury. McDougal, an award-winning journalist and runner himself, set out to understand the secrets of the Tarahumara tribe. This fast-paced story full of humor and adventure has become a 'must read' classic, in running and ultra-endurance communities.

The Complete Book of Running by James Fixx
(training/motivation/running)

Fixx's book is a favorite in the running
community. Written in 1977, this book is like
a running encyclopedia. Fixx discusses all
aspects of running from the physical gains to
the psychological benefits, such as increase
in self-esteem, the runner's "high", and
improved ability to manage everyday stress –
which, let's face it we could all use.

Find a Way by Diana Nyad
(memoir/inspirational/endurance swimmer)

This is the compelling story of Diana Nyad
who at sixty-four years young became the
first person to swim between Cuba and the
Florida Keys – with no shark cage. In her
book Nyad provides an honest account of her
life from the challenges of her childhood,
through losses, heartbreak, and the triumph
of achieving her lifelong dream after five
grueling   attempts   at   this   formidable
crossing. The message Nyad sends loud and
clear is the importance of accountability,
compassion, and the ability to face your fears
and never ever giving up on your passion no
matter how old you are or what life throws
your way.

Finding Ultra by Rich Roll
(memoir/inspirational/tri-athlete)

> *Finding Ultra* is the personal account of one man's journey from midlife crisis to ultra-endurance athlete. In his book, Roll narrates his personal struggles through alcoholism, depression, and bad relationships to a remarkable level of health, wellness, and endurance.

On Fire by John O'Leary
(memoir/inspirational)

> This book is the compelling story of John O'Leary. When John was nine years old he was involved in a house fire which almost took his life. Somehow John survived and recovered from the burns that covered almost 100% of his body. O'Leary, who is now a speaker and author, shares his incredible story of survival, courage, and strength with others in the hope that he can inspire people to live life to their fullest potential.

One Man's Mountains by Tom Patey
(memoir/adventure/mountaineer)

> This is a classic in mountaineering literature. Heralded as a celebration and memorial to "one of Britain's most charismatic and brilliant climbers" (Goodreads, 2019). Patey, also a doctor and a writer, was renowned for

revolutionizing winter climbing. Patey was killed in a rappelling accident off the coast of Scotland in 1970 at the age of 38. His book, published after his death, is an account of his assents in Scotland, Norway, and the Alps interwoven with his wit, endless energy for life, and the spirit of adventure.

The Grace to Race by Sister Madonna Buder
(memoir/inspirational/triathlete)

An inspiring account of a woman who, at 18 years old dedicated her life to the Catholic church, and then, later in life, was attracted to running as a way to balance mind, body, and soul. Her story takes the reader through the early days of rummaging through the Lost and Found to find shoes and clothing to run in; all the way to the present where, at 80-plus years old, Sister Madonna, as she is affectionately known, shares her message of love, faith, adversity, and perseverance – with boundless energy and a limitless spirit.

A Race Like No Other by Liz Robbins
(biography/inspirational/runner)

Robbins, a sports-writer for the *New York Times*, offers the reader an up close and personal view of this iconic New York City Marathon. Robbins basically dissects the 2007 New York Marathon minute by minute.

She covers it all from the athletes, the course, the atmosphere, and the army of volunteers and others working tirelessly to get almost forty thousand runners from the Verrazano-Narrows Bridge on Staten Island, through five diverse neighborhoods, all the way to the finish line at Central Park.

Run Gently Out There by John Morelock (training/inspirational/runner)

This book is a wonderful twist of trail running lore entwined with Morelock's love of the natural world. Morelock invites you to see running – not about time, fame, or awards; but rather it is about humility, community, and the pure joy of being out there and running for a lifetime.

The Run-Walk-Run Method by Jeff Galloway (training/motivation/runner)

Galloway was an average teenage runner turned Olympic athlete, trainer, and then *Runner's World* columnist and author of the Run-Walk-Run training program. His program is a favorite runners of all abilities, levels, and ages. Galloway's book covers topics from learning about running strategy, to mental training, to building form and technique, to problem solving when things don't go as planned.

Podcasts: Mentioned by the athletes

Tough Girl Podcast by Sarah Williams

The *Tough Girl Podcast* features conversations with inspirational female explorers, adventurers, and athletes. Ordinary women, from all walks of life, taking on big challenges.

Podcasts: Suggested – personally helpful

The Rich Roll Podcast by Rich Roll

Rich Roll is known for taking a deep dive into all things related to health, wellness, fitness, and nutrition. Get ready for some thought-provoking conversations with some of the brightest minds from a plethora of disciplines – from arts and science, to entertainment and business.

10% Happier Podcast by Dan Harris

Dan Harris, a correspondent for ABC news, had a very public panic attack on *Good Morning America*, which led him, through many twists and turns, to an unlikely relationship with meditation. In the podcast, Dan talks with a wide range guests about everything mindful and meditative.

Facebook Groups

Back of the Pack Athlete

I created this community as a way to support and encourage active, healthy lifestyles for the long haul. There's a general Facebook page and a private Facebook group dedicated to connection, inspiration, and motivation. The focus is on everyday "later-in-life" athletes who love their sport.

Homemade Wanderlust

A closed Facebook group all about sharing ideas, skills, knowledge and support about everything backpacking. All skill levels are welcome.

Running After 60 Group

A private Facebook group all about sharing ideas and support for runners who are dedicated to staying fit and active.

Runners Helping Runners

A private Facebook group where runners of all abilities can connect and share with other like-minded people.

Runners Over 50

This is a closed Facebook group all about feeling young at heart with lots of support for runners and walkers.

Trail and Ultra Running

An open Facebook community all about fun and support for trail and ultra-runners. All levels of experience and ability are welcome.

Slow Runners Club Walk/Run

A group for those who like to use the run/walk interval style as part of their running routine.

Women Who Hike

An organization whose mission is all about encouraging women to get out there in nature to explore, connect, and inspire.

YouTube Channels

Dixie's Wanderlust Homemade

A great resource for backpackers of all levels and abilities. Dixie – Jessica Mills – hiked the Appalachian Trial in 2015 and hasn't looked back. On her channel, Dixie talks about all her learnings; everything from gear to food to safety. There's a lot of helpful info.

Websites/Blogs Mentioned by the Athletes

Jackie Cobell – The Mad Swimmer –
http://madswimmer.com/jackie-cobell/

Five Rivers Metro Parks –
https://www.metroparks.org

International School of Mountaineering –
https://www.alpin-ism.com

A Time to Keep – Yvonne Entingh –
https://atimetokeep.net/guides/

TRX –
https://store.trxtraining.com/shop/workouts/

22 Too Many –
https://www.22toomany.com

Swimsuits for All –
https://www.swimsuitsforall.com

Note – I am a learner and consumer of words, books, and podcasts. Consequently, my list of resources seems to be perpetually evolving and expanding. If you would like to stay informed and connected with my latest suggestions, reviews, and resources please sign-up at backofthepackathlete.com.

———

APPENDIX

Races Mentioned

The Boston Marathon –
  https://www.baa.org

C&O Canal 100 Ultra –
  https://cocanal100.com

Friends of Mt. Tabor Park 5K –
  https://www.taborfriends.org/events

Hawaii Ironman – https://www.ironman.com

The Leadville 100 Ultra –
  https://www.leadvilleraceseries.com

The Marine Corps Marathon Ultra –
  https://www.marinemarathon.com

The Molokai 26-mile Swim –
  http://www.hawaiiswim.org

The New York City Marathon –
  https://www.nyrr.org

The Peaks to Portland Swim –
  https://fitmaine.com

The Philadelphia Marathon –
  https://philadelphiamarathon.com

The Siskiyou Outback Ultra –
  https://siskiyououtback.comte

The Sovereign Heritage 50k Trail Run –
  not available at time of writing

Umstead 100 Ultra –
https://umstead100.org

The Virginia Beach Marathon –
https://www.runrocknroll.com/Events/Virginia
-Beach

The Wineglass Marathon –
https://www.wineglassmarathon.com

Trails Mentioned

The American Discovery Trail –
https://discoverytrail.org

The Appalachian Trail –
http://www.appalachiantrail.org

The Eastern Continental Trail –
https://en.wikipedia.org/wiki/Eastern_Contine
ntal_Trail

The Long Trail –
https://en.wikipedia.org/wiki/Long_Trail

The Mountain to Sea Trail –
https://mountainstoseatrail.org

The New England National Scenic Trail –
https://newenglandtrail.org

The Ocala Trail –
https://www.fs.usda.gov/main/ocala/home

The Pacific Crest Trail –
https://www.pcta.org

———

ACKNOWLEDGEMENTS

ALTHOUGH INDEPENDENCE AND ADVOCACY are two of my highest values, gratitude is right up there with them. I have had a strong sense of independence from as early as I can remember. Of course, back then I was called 'stubborn' and 'bull headed', which I now celebrate, and frame as strong willed and independent.

My value around advocacy came later in life; emerging through lots of self-reflection, painful college assignments, and the education and training process which has informed my work as a mental health professional and a writer. There are many ways to define advocacy. To be clear, advocacy in my world is about raising awareness, supporting people, and being helpful.

I am especially grateful to all the people who took a chance on me and this book. To the athletes who, in good faith and generosity, gave their valuable time, energy, and personal insights to a complete stranger – without you this book would not exist. To Rebecca Myers, a local editor, who skillfully shaped and coached me through the first round of edits ready to hand off to Helen Baggott, editor extraordinaire.

Helen's patience and guidance is responsible for adding polish and professionalism; as a new independent author, I hit the jackpot! I could not have wished for more.

On a personal note, I am grateful for everything and everyone who has crossed my path during my years on the planet. All of it – the good, the bad, and the ugly – has shaped me and led me to this point today.

I am particularly grateful to the Champion side of the family for stepping in and providing light through the many storms. To my brother Sean. To friends, old and new; close and far away – thank-you for bringing joy, encouragement, and the occasional margarita into my life.

Last, but in no way least, is my small but mighty family; my two amazing, now adult, children – Benjamin and Miranda – who never cease to amaze me with their courage, energy, and determination. And my husband, Mark – my partner in life. Thank-you for being there and supporting for me through all the craziness; to love and be loved; to accept and be accepted is truly the greatest gift of all.

Final Words

IN WRAPPING-UP and considering my parting words I found a quote from Audrey Hepburn:

> "Nothing is impossible, the word itself says, 'I'm possible'."

Life is short, my friends… I urge you to chase your dreams – whatever they may be.

Lastly, I encourage you to connect and build community. Here are three ways you can link with me and other like-minded people:

The Website

If you want more running, hiking, backpacking related stuff go to: https://backofthepackathlete.com Sign-up for Tips, Tricks, & Reviews. Sometimes I offer free giveaways – books, bandanas and other cool stuff.

Facebook

Back of the Pack Athlete has a Facebook page and group offering people of all ages and fitness levels support, inspiration, and motivation – I basically created the community I was missing. Please join us at: https://www.facebook.com/backofpack/

Books

If you or a loved one is struggling with anxiety, grief, trauma, addiction, stroke or more then *You Are Limitless*—the next book in this series—is a must-read! Written in a similar style, it is inspired by people like Annie Crispino-Taylor (who, as you know, battled cancer), my experience with an auto-immune disorder, and other real people who courageously share their inspirational stories about hope and healing.

Also, make sure to grab your FREE copy of *A Pocket Guide to Hiking, Running & Backpacking: Safety Tips and Strategies*. Links to these books and more are in the following pages.

Finally, please feel free to connect with me directly at katechampionauthor.com, sign up for the *Author Happenings Newsletter*, check out the podcast *Living Big Mindfully*, or simply drop me a line. I'd love to hear from you.

Until next time...

READY FOR MORE INSPIRATION?

*If you or a loved one is struggling with anxiety, grief, trauma, addiction, stroke or more –
this book is a **must-read!***

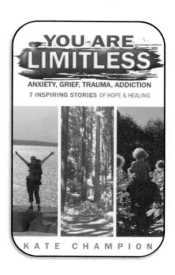

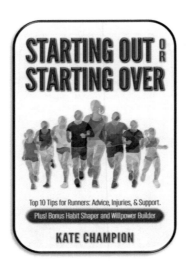

HERE'S YOUR FREE POCKET GUIDE!

Whether you are running around town, heading out for your first hike, or trekking in the backcountry – this is the book for you!

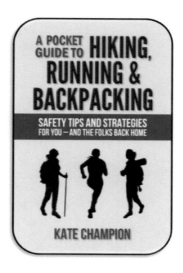

Efficient, practical, and full of tips— from first aid to trusting your gut!

Available in paperback and ebook
katechampionauthor.com
Download **FREE** today!